DEMENTIA DENIED:

One Woman's True Story of Surviving a Terminal Diagnosis & Reclaiming Her Life

***

By: S. R. HATTON

Adapted from the Memoir "Barking Mad: Recovering from Dementia" by Ginger Smith

***

Printed in the United States of America
First Printing, 2025
ISBN 979-8-9885202-8-3
Bottom Line Solutions, LLC
DBA S. R. Hatton Publishing

Contact email: SRHatton@bottomlinesolutions.net

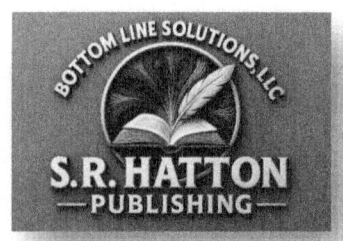

DEMENTIA DENIED

DEDICATION

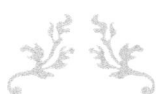

This book is dedicated to my posse, the
dementia community, and my loyal friends
and close family for their inspiration.

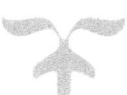

A NOTE FROM THE AUTHOR

As the author, editor, and publisher of this book, I have worked diligently to bring you the extraordinary story of **Ginger Smith** as told in her own words from her memoir "Barking Mad: Recovering from Dementia"—the traumas she endured throughout her life, her terrifying descent into dementia, and her astonishing journey back to clarity. This book is the result of countless hours spent reviewing her original memoir, emails, and video meetings, ensuring that every detail, timeline, and personal experience was captured as accurately and completely as possible.

In addition to preserving Ginger's voice and experiences, I have expanded on certain topics with extensive research, providing the most up-to-date and relevant information where it made sense to do so. Every addition was made with Ginger's full approval, with the goal of making this book not just a memoir but a valuable resource for anyone facing the complexities of dementia—whether personally or as a caregiver.

Dementia is a heavy subject, and while there is no shortage of difficult, heartbreaking moments in these pages, humor has its place, too. I firmly believe in adding lightheartedness where possible, and Ginger has her own sharp-witted, no-nonsense humor that I have done my best to preserve. You'll find it scattered throughout as a reminder that a little giggle can go a long way.

I know that dementia—and everything that comes with it—is overwhelming. That's why I've made it a priority to add as much value to this reading experience as possible. Throughout this book, you will find hyperlinks (or, if you're holding the printed version, QR codes) that will take you directly to additional resources—whether it's a deep-dive article, a downloadable guide, or a webpage filled with expert-backed information. Think of them as mini lifelines, giving you easy access to the tools and insights that might just make this journey a little less daunting. So, if something sparks your curiosity or feels especially relevant, go ahead—click (or scan), and explore. Knowledge is power, and I want to make sure you have plenty of it.

Whether you're reading this book for guidance, validation, or just a moment of relief on a tough day, I hope it brings you something meaningful. Ginger's story is one of resilience, hope, strength, and the refusal to be erased, and it has been my absolute honor to help shape it into something that can now be shared with the world.

All my best to you, ~ S. R. Hatton

A NOTE FROM GINGER

Before we dive headfirst into this medical mystery miracle memoir of mine, let me offer you a roadmap—a timeline that provides a peek at the twists, turns, and a few absurdities that have been my life.

To make your reading experience a bit easier (because trust me, even I get lost in my own medical history), I've compiled **a sequential list of major life events**—including key diagnoses, traumatic experiences, and those head-scratching moments that defy medical logic. This timeline isn't just pieced together from memory; it's the result of obsessive research, 6,500+ pages of medical records from Kaiser Permanente, countless emails, text logs, forums, journals, videos, blog posts, podcasts, medical literature reviews, and so much internet sleuthing that I probably qualify for an honorary PhD in digital forensics.

Let's just say this timeline is as accurate as humanly possible—without forcing my brain to relive every indignity more than necessary. And trust me, there's a lot to relive.

Spoiler Alert:

- There's trauma.

- There's drama.

- There's an ending so unexpected that even I still struggle to believe it.

Somewhere between being written off as "terminal" and landing an "above average" cognitive score on the MoCA test (a standardized cognitive assessment where a score of 26 or above is considered normal, 18-25 constitutes mild impairment, 11 – 17 shows moderate impairment, and 0-10 means you're in serious trouble), I managed to do the impossible: **I came back**.

Trials, Triumphs, and Really Bad Medical Luck

1937 – Born with **failure to thrive** (severely underweight and had difficulties with physical development). Exhibited **hyperkinetic behavior** (excessive activity and movement).

1941 – Suffered a violent reaction to **epinephrine** (a medication and hormone that regulates stress responses) at the dentist. Early signs of behavioral, gastrointestinal, and neurological disturbances appeared.

1942 – Developed **PTSD** (post-traumatic stress disorder) from abuse. Became regressive, fearful, and anxious.

1943 – Endured severe **parasomnias** (abnormal sleep behaviors like sleepwalking or night terrors).

1946 – First suicide attempt at age eight.

1948 – **Gaslit** (manipulated into doubting reality) by my stepfather, leading to emotional abuse, social isolation, and vulnerability.

1951 – Underwent surgery to remove a **congenitally diseased kidney** (a defect present at birth). Spent six months in the hospital.

1956 – Diagnosed with **anxiety disorder** (a condition characterized by excessive worry and fear).

1958 – Diagnosed with mental illness and escalating nerve dysfunction. Received diagnosis of **REM sleep disorder** (a condition causing disruptive or vivid dreams).

1960 – My baby, born with **osteogenesis imperfecta** (a genetic condition causing brittle bones), tragically passed away in front of me.

1962 – Behavioral and psychotic symptoms increased, including **kleptomania** (impulsive stealing) and **pica** (eating non-food substances).

1963 – Experienced **postpartum depression** (severe mood swings and depression after childbirth).

1965 – Another suicide attempt led to hospitalization.

1970 – Diagnosed with a combination of inherited brain disease and trauma-related issues.

1972 – Experienced homelessness.

1980 – Entered a live-in recovery program.

The Next Chapter of Chaos

1995 – Another suicide attempt and hospitalization.

1998 – Diagnosed with **generalized anxiety disorder** (chronic excessive worry).

2002 – Psychologists concluded my symptoms stemmed from a mix of inherited and trauma-related issues.

2004 – Relapsed into marijuana addiction after 17 years of sobriety. Entered a day rehab program. Began taking **Aricept** (*a medication for memory dysfunction*) due to suspected Alzheimer's.

2007 – Began experiencing hearing loss requiring hearing aids.

2008 – Diagnosed with **Bipolar I Disorder** (a condition causing extreme mood swings from mania to depression).

2015 – Exhibited incoherent speech and delusions. Admitted to a psychiatric hospital for suicidal ideation. Retired in December.

2016 – Presented in the ER with dementia-like features and began using a walker.

2017 – Hospitalized for complications from infected teeth. Post-surgery psychosis ensued. Family raised concerns about my mental state after noticing garbled speech and confusion.

2018 – More dementia symptoms appear, including hallucinations and tremors, leading to a neurology team referral. Neuropsychiatrist noted "exceptional cognition for age" despite clear **Parkinsonism features** (motor symptoms like tremors). MoCA score: 20/30.

2019 – After a presumptive diagnosis back in 2018 of **Frontotemporal dementia** (a rare, progressive brain disorder affecting the frontal and temporal lobes*)* and then **delusional parasitosis** (an unshakeable belief that the body is infested with parasites), I was given a differential diagnosis of "**Unspecified Dementia.**" Showed signs of **brain atrophy** (shrinkage of brain tissue) and was **aphasic** (unable to understand or express language). Emaciated after losing over 100 pounds within months. Admitted twice to a skilled nursing facility after falling eight times in one year.

2020 – Entered a board and care facility after suffering severe health deterioration. Diagnosed with possible **Lewy body dementia** (LBD) (since LBD can only definitively be diagnosed at autopsy, this was a provisional diagnosis based on symptoms and other test results). Unable to feed myself or speak coherently, I was bedbound, paranoid, hallucinating, and suffered many **UTIs** (urinary tract infections). Put in hospice with all medications discontinued except for those needed for my comfort and given approximately two weeks to live. Mysteriously and very slowly began to regain the ability to walk, talk, and think.

2021 – Returned home. Despite mild short-term memory loss, I became mostly independent in daily living activities. Began drafting my memoir.

2022 – Achieved a MoCA score of 28/30 (basically normal). Bipolar disorder was declared in full remission. Cognitive testing showed above-average function for my age.

2023 – Neurocognitive testing confirmed no dementia. Scored a perfect 30 on the MoCA.

I share this history not as a plea for sympathy but as proof that resilience can exist in the face of impossible odds. For years, I've navigated the murky waters of medical errors, misdiagnoses, and outright quackery—and if my story helps even one person avoid the pitfalls of pseudo-medical nonsense, advocate for better care, or simply feel a little less alone, then laying my life bare in these pages will have been worth it.

But let's be clear: It hasn't been all doom and gloom. Somewhere between the catastrophes, I've managed to carve out a pretty fulfilling life—proof that no matter how much junk life throws at you, a few sparkling gems can usually be found in the debris.

Before we dive in, I also want to take a moment to acknowledge Kaiser Permanente. Having been part of their system for over 40 years—both as an employee and a patient—I can confidently say they are highly respected in the industry for their focus on preventive healthcare. My publisher has put together a free download detailing exactly why I stand by that statement—if you're curious, you can check it out at this **LINK**.

Also, a quick warning: I have a tendency to ramble, nerd out over medical science, and use humor as a coping mechanism. Some of my friends and peers have lovingly teased me about how much "mind-blowingly dull medical jargon" I manage to sneak into casual conversation. My editor has done her best to keep that in check, but I make no promises.

This book is messy. It's raw, unfiltered, and unapologetically real. But if there's one thing I hope you take away from it, it's this:

Even in the darkest places, there's always a sliver of light worth holding onto.

I hope this book helps you find yours.

With warm regards,

Ginger Smith

Contents

PREFACE

My grandson, Josh, recently showed me a video he had taken during one of the darkest, most surreal moments of my life. In it, I sat in the passenger seat of a car, my words tangled in delusion as I earnestly explained that an ER doctor had just removed a piece of plastic from my mouth that had been sewn in to keep me from barking. The recording started just after the real spectacle—because moments earlier, I had been barking like a dog. And not just any dog—Hitler's German Shepherd.

Yes, you read that correctly.

Josh, handling it with a grace beyond his years, quietly pulled out his phone and hit 'record.' No mockery, no judgment—just discreet documentation of a moment my family would have otherwise struggled to explain. Watching it now, I can see it for what it was: tragic, absurd, and terrifying proof of just how far I had fallen.

Doctors were calling it **"irreversible dementia."** My loved ones were told to prepare for the inevitable.

Yet here I am, years later, writing this book.

How did I find my way back? That question lingers in my mind—and I imagine it's why you're here. This memoir is my attempt to unravel the mystery of how I traveled through the depths of dementia and somehow returned, a phenomenon that still baffles my doctors. One of them recently called it a "rare, complete recovery from dementia"—though from the look on his face, I might as well have been a lab rat that had gone rogue.

I spent years working as a speech-language pathologist, working with neurology pros at Stanford University Medical Hospital and training physicians at UCSF and Stanford to diagnose and treat communication and cognitive disorders. My job involved untangling complex medical mysteries, advocating for my patients, and training other professionals to do the same.

The irony of becoming a medical anomaly myself is not lost on me. I went from respected clinician to **"terminal dementia patient"** in nearly the blink of an eye—only to claw my way back from the depths of neurocognitive decline, much to the bewilderment of the same system that had written me off.

This book is a little bit of everything—part detective novel, part medical misadventure, part dark comedy, and part unapologetic exposé. A friend once jokingly called it my "oughtography," but honestly, I think *"TMI-ography"* might be more fitting—and you'll soon see why. I've pulled together an authentic and compelling narrative, one that doesn't hold back on the raw, the ridiculous, or the downright unbelievable.

It's for those who have been misdiagnosed, overmedicated, gaslit, dismissed, abandoned, or left to languish in facilities where "care" is little more than a checkbox on a form. And it's for anyone who's ever wondered if maybe, just maybe, *our healthcare system was put together by amateurs*.

Through it all, I've learned that life has a twisted sense of humor. And sometimes, the only way to survive the absurdity is to laugh right along with it.

****

If you're curious (or just in need of a good chuckle at my expense), you can check out an excerpt of the infamous *"barking like a dog"* video by scanning the QR code below. Let me set the scene for you: My grandsons and my oldest son, Ty, were bringing me home from yet another emergency room visit when, out of nowhere, I started *barking at them*—like a dog. But I didn't stop there. Oh no. I then declared, with absolute conviction, that I was Hitler's German Shepherd.

At that point, Josh decided this moment needed to be immortalized because, let's be honest, who would believe them otherwise? So, he pulled out his phone and started recording. The video picks up right after my big announcement, capturing my latest dementia-fueled antics. It's mostly audio (we were driving at night, so the lighting wasn't great in the car), but trust me— the sound alone is enough.

If you're unfamiliar with them, here are the steps to using QR codes:

1. **Get Your Phone Ready**: Grab your smartphone. Most phones today, like iPhones or Androids, can scan QR codes without needing extra apps, but we'll cover that too.

2. **Open the Camera**: Open the camera app on your phone, just like you're about to take a picture. Point the camera at the QR code so it's in the frame. Make sure the whole square fits on your screen and it's not too blurry.

3. **Look for a Pop-Up**: If your phone recognizes the QR code, a little notification or link will pop up on the screen. For example, on an iPhone, you might see a yellow link box, or on an Android, a small banner might appear. Tap it! It'll take you to whatever the QR code is linked to, like a website or a video.

4. **No Pop-Up? Try This**: If nothing happens, your phone might need a little help. Some phones don't auto-scan QR codes with the camera. In that case, download a free QR code reader app from the App Store (iPhone) or Google Play Store (Android). Open the app, point it at the QR code, and it'll do the rest.

ACKNOWLEDGEMENTS

This book would not have been possible without the unwavering support, encouragement, and kindness of so many incredible people. I am truly blessed to have what I call *my Posse*—the friends and community members who have lifted me up, stood by my side, and reminded me that I am never alone.

To my editor and publisher, **Shanlynn (S. R. Hatton)**—I owe you the highest respect and deepest gratitude for believing in my story and helping bring it to life.

To my incredible SLP friends—**Katherine, Tiffany, and my bestie, Pam**—thank you for keeping me grounded in the work we love.

From *The Villages*, my gratitude to **Theresa, Ekatarina, Beverly, Carolyn, and Erica** for your kindness and support.

To the wonderful women of the **Fair Oaks Senior Center—Rachel and Patricia**—your friendship has meant the world to me.

To the *Friendly Voices* who have lifted my spirits—**Judith and Lynn**—thank you for always being there.

To my incredible support network in the **dementia community**—**Laurie, Mark, Creeky, and Kathleen from DAA** (*Dementia Action Alliance*), as well as **Kate from DAI** (*Dementia Alliance International*)—your advocacy and resilience inspire me daily.

To my helpful friends—**Matt at SVdP Society,** and **Janice, Victoria, Denice, Jennifer, and Alton**—thank you for showing up when I needed you most.

To the remarkable **LAG Crusaders—Deborah, Julie, Mary, Jeanie, and Pauline**—thank you for your efforts and unwavering support.

To **Tess** from *Peninsula Family Service*—your kindness has made such a difference, and to **Maria**, my very first volunteer, thank you for believing in me.

To my **LifeRing** friends—**Gail, Ed, Jim, and Dave**—thank you for walking this path with me, and to **JoAnne**, with special love for your recovery.

To **Anne Jackson**, PhD—You quite literally changed my life with your insights and encouragement.

To **Zahida**, who messages me every day, and **Ginny**, whose friendship knows no bounds—you both have brightened my days in ways you'll never know.

To my *NextDoor* special angels, **The Ferri Family—Dana, Sean, and Nico**—your kindness is nothing short of extraordinary.

And, of course, to my beloved **family—Ty, Tanya, Shawn, Jeremy, Cody, and Josh**—I love you beyond words.

With loving thoughts to my sister, **Sandy**, and special thanks to **Chris** for keeping us connected through Zoom.

Each of you has played a role in my journey, whether through support, encouragement, laughter, or simply being there when I needed it most. I am forever grateful.

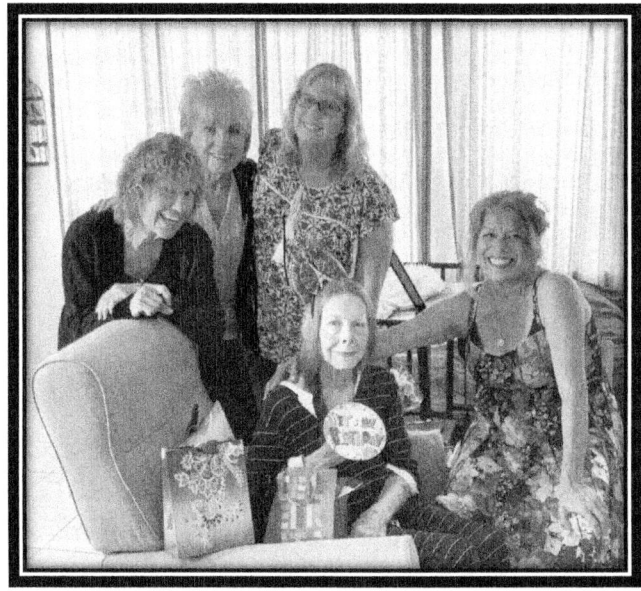

Me & my Posse after I came home from hospice

INTRODUCTION

I feel it's important to tell you about a few more things before you start reading—this isn't just a memoir. It's also a bit of a survival guide stitched together with grit, a little humor, and the hard-won wisdom of someone who has walked through nearly every fire life could light. It isn't just about surviving but about rebuilding, reinventing, and reclaiming yourself, no matter how broken the pieces seem.

In these pages, you'll meet me first as a young girl navigating a traumatic world that offered few safe places. My childhood taught me two essential skills: how to stand my ground and how to laugh when nothing else made sense. That humor became my lifeline, a tool I carried into adulthood as I faced addiction, mental health struggles, and the challenges of building a career in speech-language pathology—guiding others to find their voices even as I struggled to hold onto my own.

Then came the unexpected diagnosis that changed everything.

Neurocognitive disorders, including **Frontotemporal** and **Lewy body dementia**, entered the picture. Doctors told me it was *terminal*. My world became one of hallucinations, paranoia, and care facilities where I was eventually labeled *"end-stage."* It was a descent into a medical mystery, a test of endurance in ways I couldn't have imagined.

But here's the unexpected and downright baffling twist: ***I didn't die***.

Despite every prediction, I clawed my way back—leaving doctors puzzled and skeptics questioning how something like this could even be possible.

Today, I am home, and as independent as I can be at the age of nearly 88 with activities of daily living. I am functional, and I am sharing this story to shed light on the hidden battles of dementia: trauma, misdiagnosis, overmedication, and a healthcare system that too often gets it wrong.

But that's not all.

I've also proudly donned my pioneer hat (it's metaphorical, but let's pretend it's fabulous) to expose medical pseudoscience frauds—those charming con artists who could gaslight a lighthouse. These frauds prey on the vulnerable, peddling phony cures and false hope to desperate people. I've seen the damage they cause, and part of my mission is to drag their shady tactics into the spotlight.

And finally, I'll explore the medical mystery of my own survival—because, frankly, even I don't fully understand it. I have theories, and I'll break them down for you, drawing from my background in neurology, speech pathology, and lived experience.

This memoir isn't just a collection of stories, it's a call to action for anyone who is willing to join me.

I hope it sparks research, raises awareness, and challenges the litany of medical missteps that plague dementia care: **iatrogenic errors** (harm caused by medical treatment), ineffective therapies, ageist stereotypes, and the profiteers who exploit the sick and elderly.

And so, we begin—not with the miraculous twist you may be eager to unravel, but with the struggles that shaped the person I am today—because resilience isn't something you're simply born with, it's something you build, piece by piece, in the midst of chaos, hardship, and survival.

CHAPTER 1: BORN INTO PRIVILEGE, RAISED IN CHAOS

On the surface, my life began with all the hallmarks of privilege and promise—born into an upper-class home in Berkeley, California, with a charmed lineage and parents who seemed, at least on paper, like they were scripted for a storybook beginning.

My father was a living contradiction—a brilliant, handsome, charismatic war hero, and supposedly, at the time, had the highest IQ in the state. Which, in California terms, probably meant he could do advanced calculus while surfing.

He had been a yell leader at UC Berkeley (which, for the uninitiated, is a spirited male cheerleader responsible for leading chants and rallying the crowd) before becoming the youngest district attorney ever elected in California. The world was at his feet.

But that world came with demons.

PTSD—what they called "shell shock" back then—twisted him into someone unrecognizable. Alcoholism swallowed him whole.

What began as a meteoric rise ended in utter collapse.

He became homeless.

Or, as he put it in the few letters he managed to send me later in life, he became a "hobo."

(I actually prefer his term—it has a certain panache compared to today's sterile "unhoused.")

My father was a man who enlisted in a war he didn't have to fight. He had a newborn at home and a wife who needed him, yet he still went.

He survived the Battle of the Bulge, was wounded numerous times, and collected multiple Purple Hearts—physical proof that he had given his body and mind to war, piece by piece, until there was nothing left to salvage.

He died in his early 40s, his body ravaged by cirrhosis of the liver, leaving behind a legacy of brilliance, brokenness, and heartbreak.

A Mother Caught in the Storm

My mother, the quintessential society girl, was beautiful, sweet, and entirely unprepared for the chaos she married into.

She had no idea how to handle a violent, self-destructive alcoholic or a sickly, difficult child (me).

So, my care fell largely to my maternal grandmother, a former hospital administrator and no-nonsense woman of extraordinary competence who had once navigated the pandemonium of the 1906 earthquake.

She met my maternal grandfather, the director of volunteers for the local fire company, in the aftermath of that disaster. Together, they revolutionized emergency medical care, introducing San Francisco's first engine-powered ambulance—a lifesaving innovation that undoubtedly saved countless lives.

My grandfather, however, did not fare so well himself.

In 1929, he was found dead in his garage—carbon monoxide poisoning.

For decades, I was fed a sanitized version of the story—it was a tragic accident, a misunderstanding, a slip-up with the car running.

It wasn't until my 40s that I overheard the real truth: he had taken his own life.

You would think that the timing of his death—right at the start of the Great Depression—would've been a flashing neon clue. But, as it turns out, family secrets thrive on convenient omissions.

A Childhood of Exile

My early years were marked by a pattern of abandonment—boarding schools, summer camps, and whatever else kept me at a comfortable distance from home.

It was a year-round exile, one that made me self-reliant to a fault, but also untethered, unsure of where I truly belonged.

My mother and I grew closer later in life, but our journey toward healing came too late—by the time we found our deepest connection, she was dying.

Throat cancer.

In the end, she passed away in my arms—our final years together were bittersweet, filled with love, pain, and the kind of unspoken apologies that only come when it's too late to rewrite the past.

When Trauma Came Knocking

But let's rewind to the most harrowing chapter of my early life.

The day my father tried to kill me.

I was just a child, but I remember it with terrifying clarity—the moment my paternal grandfather caught him in the act, the chaos that erupted, the realization that I was now old enough to talk coherently and expose what he had been doing to me.

The sexual abuse.

That was the real reason he wanted me gone.

That day, he was forcibly removed from our home.

It was the last time I ever saw him—except for one strange, fleeting moment years later.

The Man on the Hill

I was at boarding school, standing on a hill, looking down at a handsome man in an Army uniform.

Something in me stirred.

Could that be my father?

I ran down the hill, desperate to reach him, to confirm what my heart already knew.

But before I got there, the school principal intercepted me—and sent him away.

And just like that, he was gone.

I never saw him again.

Letters from a Ghost

He wrote me letters, though.

Affectionate letters.

A little *too* affectionate.

In hindsight, the way he described me—calling me "charming," painting images of the life he lived as a wanderer, sharing campfires and food with fellow "hobos"—was deeply unsettling.

Even now, I wonder if my own relentless crusading spirit—this compulsion to help the lost and forgotten—comes from him, from his self-proclaimed mission to find meaning among the dispossessed.

But his legacy was a tangled mess of love and destruction.

And my own survival?

I believe it's a testament to the fact that I was rescued from him before it was too late.

The Forbidden Goodbye

Years later, when he lay dying of liver failure, I wasn't allowed to visit.

My mother and stepfather deemed me "too sensitive" to handle it.

But the truth is, I probably would have been just fine.

It wasn't rage that filled me when I thought of him.

Not even hatred.

Just an endless, aching sadness—a grief not for who he was, but for who he could have been.

For the father I never had.

For the man he might have been if war and alcohol hadn't destroyed him.

For the story that was over before I ever had a chance to rewrite it.

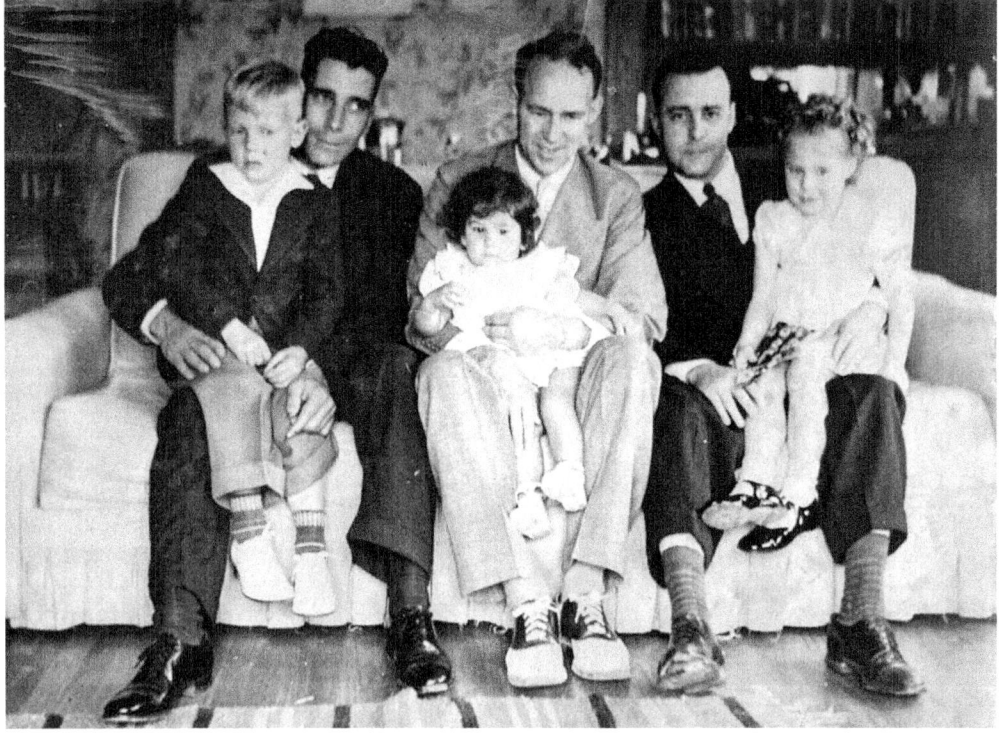

Me & my Dad (far right) with my Uncles & Cousins

CHAPTER 2: PRAYERS & PUNISHMENT

By the age of six, I had already decided that faith healing wasn't for me—though my mother clearly had other plans. And so began my forced spiritual enlightenment, delivered via a scenic yet emotionally scarring tour of religious boarding schools.

The first stop on this soul-purifying journey was Children's Christian Science Country School, a place that looked straight out of a storybook—quaint cobblestone paths, a grand carriage house, and dormitories that screamed "future trauma memoir." Their approach to health? Healing through prayer rather than medical intervention. Sounds lovely in theory—until you're the one writhing in pain.

The school also embraced what I can only assume was a trend among cruel 20th-century educators: "spartan settings." Apparently, if deprivation was good enough for the offspring of European royalty, it was certainly good enough for a sickly child like me. No comfort, no warmth—just a disciplinary program wrapped in a neat little package of forced manual labor.

For example, I spent my summer days picking apricots in the fields (a "strict disciplinary program" disguised as agricultural servitude). Looking back, I wonder if those pesticide-drenched fruits were sowing more than just discipline—recent research has linked pesticide exposure to neurodegenerative diseases like Parkinson's. So, perhaps they were also handing out a free degenerative illness with every basket.

But I wasn't just an overworked child laborer, I was also a walking medical disaster. I was born with severe kidney disease, which meant my face was constantly swollen and jaundiced, my body bloated from fluid retention, and my bladder about as reliable as an overfilled water balloon.

I was a hormonal, sickly child who smelled like a urinal, making me a prime target for bullies. Bed-wetting was an almost nightly occurrence, and as if the embarrassment of that wasn't enough, discipline for it involved public humiliation and, occasionally, a beating with a wooden hanger.

And when my kidneys weren't actively torturing me, the school's medieval medical practices stepped in to pick up the slack. At one point, my legs became covered in painful boils, which the school's headmistress scraped off—without anesthetic—as though she were trying to win a prize for Most Misguided Medical Practitioner.

Suicide Doors

By the time I was eight years old, I had officially reached my breaking point. After enduring the sexual abuse at home, this new life of bottomless bullying and relentless physical pain became unbearable, and so I did what any desperate child might do: I tried to end it all.

My method? I threw myself out of a moving car. And not just any car—one with rear-hinged "suicide doors" (how poetic). I landed on the gravel, which embedded itself into my knees, and spent months bedridden while every last jagged piece was painstakingly picked from my skin.

At the time, I had no conscious memory of why I had done it. I repressed it so deeply that I only uncovered the truth while writing this memoir. The act of memory suppression, or **dissociative amnesia** (the inability to recall traumatic events), is controversial, even among scientists.

I had spent decades dismissing "recovered memories" as pseudo-science, yet here they were—crystal clear and gut-wrenching. And like it or not, the research supports it: early childhood trauma, particularly sexual abuse, increases the risk of suicide. But knowing that doesn't make it any easier to process.

The Horse That Saved Me—Until She Didn't

In the chaos of my childhood, there was one bright spot: Ginger, the fiery sorrel horse my parents bought me. She was my refuge, my sanctuary. She was also completely unrideable for anyone but me—we shared an understanding, a silent agreement that in a world that made no sense, we had each other.

Naturally, in what would become a recurring theme of my life, my parents sold her.

I was devastated—and furious in a way only a ten-year-old can be. So, I did the only thing within my power to reclaim some control: I changed my name.

Carol was gone. *Ginger* was born.

My parents objected, of course, but stubbornness is one of my defining traits. From that moment on, Ginger became my identity, my badge of defiance, and the name I have carried ever since.

The Power of Pretending

At some point, I learned that manipulation was survival. I had to hide the constant physical agony of my undiagnosed kidney disease, the shame of my bedwetting, and the weight of abuse that threatened to crush me. I got good at playing whatever role I needed to:

- I lied.
- I shoplifted.
- I found ways to justify my worst behavior.

But at the same time, I threw myself into helping others, desperate to balance the scales—a trait that would follow me into adulthood as a speech therapist and lifelong volunteer. Was I seeking redemption or recognition? Probably both.

Still, there were small glimpses of light in the darkness:

- Movies like *South Pacific*, *Showboat*, and *Inherit the Wind* offered me an escape into a world that felt bigger than my suffering.
- My kind, patient grandmother became my emotional anchor during the few holidays I was allowed away from school.
- Books, stories, and plays became my obsession, my way of imagining something greater than my bleak reality.

Burning It All Down—Literally

As if my time at Christian Science school hadn't been traumatic enough, the building burned to the ground before I left.

I'd love to say this felt like poetic justice, but mostly, I remember lying in the infirmary—completely forgotten—because I couldn't walk. This was shortly after I had badly damaged my legs from my suicide attempt, and in the chaos of evacuation, apparently, nobody thought to count all the students.

At the last minute, someone realized I was missing and dragged me out. My family still jokes that my school had to burn before they would finally let me graduate.

And yet, despite everything, I had been an excellent student. Turns out, trauma makes you resourceful.

Out of the Fire & into the Frying Pan of Faith

After Christian Science school had failed to heal me—or protect me from relentless suffering—I was shipped off to Sacred Heart Convent, an elite boarding school in Menlo Park. The grand first floor, draped in rich tapestries and jeweled decor, created the illusion of refinement and grace, but upstairs, in the cold, sparse dormitories, reality was far less glamorous.

The school nurse had a special talent for making bad situations worse. Instead of investigating my constant pain, she decided the solution was endless enemas, a treatment plan that made about as much sense as leech therapy. My undiagnosed kidney disease continued to wreak havoc on my body, but rather than receive medical attention, I was left to endure the suffering with no explanation.

Despite this, I found small victories. I shone in school plays, landing lead roles and momentarily escaping into other identities. I also made it my mission to outscore the Catholics in catechism class—an entirely unnecessary feat, but one I took great pride in. My theatrics, however, weren't always welcome. One morning, desperate to avoid mass, I faked fainting. The nuns weren't amused.

My weight, a combination of stress eating and my illness, also made me a target. One day, the head nun summoned me to her office. For a brief moment, I thought I might be receiving some kind of honor. Instead, she bluntly informed me that I had gotten too fat for my uniform and needed new clothes. Whatever shred of self-esteem I had left took another hit.

By my final year there, I slipped into what I now think of as my "undercover boy" phase—binding my breasts, speaking in a low voice, and hiding beneath a hat. At the time, I didn't fully understand why I was doing it, but looking back, it was an attempt to make myself invisible. A way to reject the body that had betrayed me so many times before. The strangest part? ***No one noticed***. Not my teachers, not my classmates—no one.

The Angst of High School

Leaving the knuckle-whacking nuns behind and joining San Mateo High School was merely a change in geography, not circumstance. I still had no friends, no social life, and a lineup of psychological demons keeping me company, so I filled my time babysitting.

One of my regular jobs was for a neighbor who owned the only TV in the area. I would stay late, watching whatever was on after the kids were asleep. That's exactly what I was doing the night my entire life changed.

I had spent years enduring pain so severe it felt like being electrocuted from the inside. Up to that point, I hadn't realized it wasn't *normal* to live in constant agony, thanks to **uremic neuropathy** (nerve damage caused by kidney failure). But I had been told it was "all in my head"—that I was "showboating," or even a hypochondriac. So, I learned to hide it, assuming everyone must feel this way and that I was simply weaker than the rest.

On that particular night, I was curled up in front of the TV watching *Dragnet*. Then, without warning, the pain escalated past anything I had ever known. It was unbearable, like my entire body was tearing apart from the inside. Assuming I could privately indulge in my breakdown without an audience, I collapsed onto the floor, writhing, unable to stop the violent sobs escaping my throat.

I didn't hear the door open. I had no idea my neighbor had returned early until I saw his face—a mix of horror and urgency. And fate, for once, had impeccable timing because he wasn't just my neighbor.

He was a doctor.

Within minutes, he rushed me to the hospital. I don't remember much except being wheeled into surgery. When I woke up, my extra kidney—the cause of my years of suffering—was finally gone.

Oh, and as a casual side note, they also informed me—ever so nonchalantly—that I had *died* on the operating table. Just a little extra trauma to add to the mix at that still-young-and-impressionable age.

For years, I had no idea what had actually been done to me. All I was told was that they had operated on my left kidney. It wasn't until much later—during an unrelated ultrasound—that a technician casually mentioned, "Oh, you had an extra kidney removed." Without missing a beat, I quipped, "Oh? Was it a boy or a girl?"

The Road to Recovery (With a Slight Detour Through Hell)

The surgery may have saved my life, but recovery was another beast entirely. Six months in the hospital meant enduring excruciating bladder irrigations and becoming a medical curiosity. Apparently, I was such a "rare case" that every curious resident in the building needed a front-row seat to examine my most private areas.

As if that wasn't degrading enough, while lying on a gurney awaiting yet another procedure, I was sexually assaulted by a hospital orderly who had posed as a doctor. My body, once again, had been reduced to something for others to use, examine, and exploit.

Physically, I was healing. Emotionally, I was unraveling. But even then, I clung to the one thing that had always saved me—my bawdy and twisted sense of humor. Because sometimes, the only way to survive the unthinkable is to laugh in its face.

My parents were deeply apologetic for all the years they had ignored my suffering, but I didn't blame them. They had done their best, navigating a world that had failed us both. To make up for everything, they bought me a St. Bernard puppy. I named him Brandy, and he became my greatest source of comfort.

By the time I was discharged from the hospital, I wasn't the same person. I was thinner, healthier, and determined to make up for lost time.

A New Life, A Familiar Darkness

Back at San Mateo High, I thrived. I excelled academically, won speaking contests, and even found myself dancing with the governor during a trip to the State Capitol. I was elected to a school office, started dating the class president, and for the first time, it looked like I was becoming the girl I had always wanted to be.

But my demons didn't disappear.

I ran away from home constantly, slipping out into the night, hoping someone would notice—hoping someone would care enough to come after me. But no one ever did. I'd wander the streets, sometimes sleeping in strangers' cars, before eventually returning home, exhausted and ashamed that no one had missed me.

The Theater (And the Power of a Well-Timed Meltdown)

If there was one place I could always count on feeling seen, it was on stage.

I took on lead roles in nearly every school play, my love of performance flourishing into a kind of emotional survival tactic. I also quickly realized that if I so much as *whispered* about feeling unwell, an entire production crew would leap into action.

My ability to play the fragile, tragic heroine was unparalleled.

For a while, I was the perfect student—well-behaved, high-achieving, adored. Then, during one fateful dress rehearsal, something inside me just *snapped*. Maybe it was the pressure, maybe it was sheer exhaustion, or maybe I was just tired of being perfect. Whatever the reason, I got kicked out of the play.

Humiliated, I stormed out in a melodramatic flourish worthy of an Oscar. That tantrum landed me in detention, where I made a groundbreaking discovery: Detention was where all the cute bad boys were hiding.

Had I known that earlier, I might have started acting out much sooner.

A Grandmother's Love Stops My Self-Destruction

Through it all, my grandmother remained my anchor. She had moved all the way from Napa to San Mateo, settling into an apartment nearby and offering me a place of stability and unconditional love.

It was through her that I finally found the strength to stop the self-harm that had quietly consumed me for years.

Cutting, burning—I had secretly been doing it all, believing that the only way to release the pain inside me was to carve it out of my own skin. It wasn't until much later in life that I realized how many trauma survivors do the same.

A Step Too Far

As if the school atmosphere wasn't enough, my stepfather—a deacon in the church—was there to make sure my torment didn't take a day off.

To be clear, he never laid a hand on me physically, nor did he abuse me in the way my father had, but he excelled in emotional cruelty like it was an Olympic sport. His lectures about my heathen ways could last an hour or more, masterpieces of guilt and shame woven together with fire-and-brimstone flair. According to him, I was destined for hell, which, if I'm being honest, sounded only slightly worse than spending another hour in his company.

Public humiliation was his forte. He had a way of targeting my deepest vulnerabilities, finding the exact thing that would make me feel small, exposed, or unworthy. If I pushed back? That was just proof of my manipulative nature. If I refused to convert to his brand of faith? I was being histrionic—dramatic, theatrical, attention-seeking. And my kidney disease? Pure fabrication. Because clearly, my uremic neuropathy was just a cry for attention.

He had another skill, one I didn't have a name for back then, but now I know it well: gaslighting.

Gaslighting is a psychological abuse tactic designed to warp reality, to make you doubt your own memories, perceptions, and even sanity. If a gaslighter tells you the sky is green and you argue it's blue, they'll convince you you're colorblind. Or worse, delusional. Their ultimate goal is to exert control by discrediting you until you no longer trust yourself. And my stepfather was a master at it.

For years, he made me feel crazy. If I contradicted him, I was unstable. If I expressed pain, I was exaggerating. If I challenged his beliefs, I was rebellious and sinful. No matter what I did, I was always wrong. And when you're young and vulnerable, that kind of manipulation seeps into your bones.

The Long Road to Understanding

Despite my intense hatred for him as a child, I recognize now that he was a man battling his own demons. That doesn't excuse what he did, but it helps explain why he was so determined to break me. He wanted control in a world that had none. He wanted certainty in a life that was unpredictable. And in his mind, if he could mold me into his version of "righteous," then he had won.

It took years of therapy and painful introspection, but eventually, I came to see the full picture. He was a deeply flawed man, but in his own way, he did try to be a good stepfather. We managed to reach a fragile peace in my adulthood. And though I never fully forgave him, I at least came to understand him.

The Shock of Validation

For years, I buried most of these memories, half-convinced I had imagined them. I knew what I had endured at school, I knew the pain was real, but part of me always wondered:

Had I made it worse in my mind? Had I exaggerated? Had time distorted the truth?

And then, one day, I got my answer.

My cousin, who had also survived that boarding school, confirmed it all. She had witnessed it firsthand. The abuse and discipline tactics I had questioned, every horror I had tried to forget—she remembered it too.

I should have felt validated. Instead, it made everything worse. Because now I knew for certain that it hadn't just been "bad memories" or "childhood exaggeration." It had been real.

And I probably owe her a therapy session or two for dredging it all back up.

Survival Isn't Pretty, But It's Mine

If sharing my story convinces even one parent to think twice before sending their child to a religious boarding school, or at the very least, one that substitutes abuse for medical care, then reliving these moments will have been worth it.

Through it all, I developed a kind of Teflon resilience—not the polished, inspirational kind, but the stubborn, messy kind that gets you through the worst.

Life handed me some of the darkest moments imaginable.

But I'm still here.

Still standing.

Still telling my story.

And still answering to the name I chose for myself: Ginger.

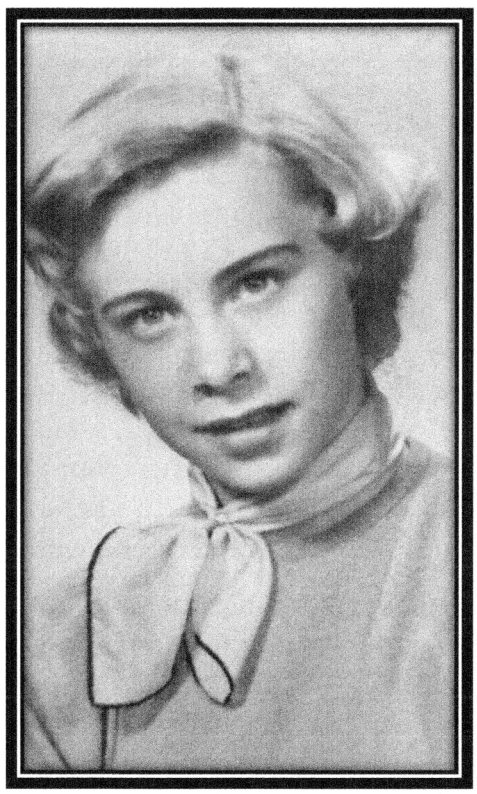

My High School photo (circa 1954)

CHAPTER 3: WHEN THE PAST HAUNTS THE PRESENT

Before diving further into the tangled mess that is my life story, it's important to highlight four key psychological concepts that have, for better or worse, shaped the way my brain has operated for decades: **child sexual abuse (CSA), gaslighting, core-sounding, and rejection-sensitive dysphoria (RSD).** These aren't just academic terms—they're the very foundations of my trauma, the invisible strings that pulled me toward emotional instability, self-destruction, and, ultimately, survival.

For years, I wrestled with the fallout of these forces without understanding how they worked together, how they rewired my brain, and how they set the stage for a long, slow cognitive and physical breakdown that would take years to unravel.

If trauma is a puzzle, these are the corner pieces.

Child Sexual Abuse (CSA): The Unseen Scars

CSA is a term clinical researchers use to describe any sexual activity between a child and an adult or older adolescent—everything from physical contact to exposure to pornography. In reality, CSA is an earthquake that shakes the foundation of a child's sense of safety and self-worth, leaving cracks that widen over time.

The effects don't fade when the abuse stops. Instead, they metastasize into a lifetime of psychological landmines—depression, anxiety, PTSD, and relationship dysfunction. Survivors like me often struggle with trust, body image, and a gnawing sense that something fundamental was taken from them before they even had the language to understand what it was.

But the damage isn't just emotional. Research has shown that survivors of CSA are more likely to suffer from chronic pain, gastrointestinal disorders, heart disease, and obesity (Jeglic, 2021). It's as if the body, unable to process what happened, keeps trying to store the trauma somewhere—stashing it in nerve endings, muscle tension, and gut imbalances until it finally explodes in a full-blown health crisis. In my case, it shaped everything: how I saw myself, how I interacted with the world, and how I would later unravel.

Gaslighting: Warping Reality

If CSA is the earthquake, gaslighting is the aftershock that ensures you never quite trust the ground beneath you again.

Gaslighting is a form of psychological manipulation where an abuser makes the victim question their reality—turning certainty into confusion and self-confidence into self-doubt (Engel, 2024). When gaslighting is sustained over time, it chips away at a person's ability to trust their own mind. And once you stop trusting yourself, you become dependent on the very people distorting your reality.

I was gaslit by my family, by school authorities, and later, even in skilled nursing facilities (SNFs). My kidney pain wasn't real, I was just being dramatic. My father wasn't trying to kill me, I was exaggerating. My memories of abuse were false, a figment of an overactive imagination. Every time I tried to assert my truth, someone was there to tell me I was wrong.

Imagine being a computer with a hacked hard drive—files corrupted, system overridden, commands no longer your own. That was my brain. By the time I reached adulthood, I second-guessed everything about myself. Did I actually feel pain, or was I imagining it? Did I deserve the things that happened to me? Was I really as manipulative as they said? The only thing I knew for sure was that I didn't know *anything* for sure.

Core-Sounding: The Echoes of Childhood

There's a psychological theory that our earliest experiences create the "core sound" that reverberates throughout our entire lives. It's the emotional undertone, the background noise that shapes how we see the world and ourselves.

For children raised in love, that sound might be a symphony of safety, support, and self-worth. For those of us who grew up in trauma, it's more like a broken record of fear, rejection, and pain, skipping on the same note over and over again.

Early interactions with parents, caregivers, and peers play a pivotal role in constructing the brain's architecture. Positive engagements can lead to robust mental health, while negative or inconsistent interactions may result in vulnerabilities. As noted by the Center on the Developing Child at Harvard University, early experiences significantly influence the developing brain's architecture (*INBrief: Early Childhood Mental Health*, 2020).

My core sound was shaped before I even had language. The gaslighting about my kidney disease, the constant bullying, the endless days spent alone without a single friend, the punishments, the beatings, the abuse. This was my foundation. Imagine trying to build a house when all you've got are flimsy walls, a rotting floor, and nails made of Jell-O. That was my emotional structure—wobbly, fragile, and completely unfit for long-term survival.

Rejection-Sensitive Dysphoria: The Sting of Perceived Rejection

Rejection-Sensitive Dysphoria (RSD) is like having an emotional amplifier permanently set to high—every perceived or actual rejection, criticism, or failure hits with an intensity that can feel overwhelming.

Individuals with RSD don't just feel disappointment; they experience emotional pain so deeply that it can lead to avoidance of situations where rejection might occur. This heightened sensitivity often results in withdrawing from social interactions, hesitating to take risks, or even struggling with self-worth.

They too often become chronic people-pleasers, bending over backward to make sure they're never seen as a burden. Or they withdraw entirely, avoiding situations where they might fail. I did both.

Though commonly associated with ADHD, RSD can also occur independently, making emotional regulation a challenge. The Cleveland Clinic describes RSD as a condition that disrupts a person's ability to manage emotional responses to perceived failure or rejection (*Rejection Sensitive Dysphoria (RSD)*, 2024).

Imagine an overactive smoke alarm that blares at the slightest hint of smoke—whether it's a raging fire or just burnt toast. That's how RSD functions in the brain, setting off intense reactions even when the actual threat is minimal.

Like Planting Seeds in Poisoned Soil

The more research I've done in recent years, the clearer it's become: adverse childhood experiences don't just leave emotional scars; they set off long-term health crises.

The trauma I experienced wasn't just something I had to "get over." It was actively rewiring my brain, altering my stress response, my immune system, and even my cognitive abilities. I wasn't just shaped by my past—I was trapped in it.

For years, I tried to make sense of why my brain and body were falling apart. And now I understand: trauma doesn't just live in memories. It lives in the body, in the cells, in the way the nervous system learns to brace for impact long after the danger is gone.

Trauma hasn't just been a few chapters in my life story—it's been the headliner in a long-running, critically unacclaimed drama.

The plot twists? Incest. My father trying to kill me. A dozen hospitalizations. A near-death experience.

If there were awards for surviving early-life chaos, I'd at least be nominated.

Traumas of the Fifth Kind

Once I reached adulthood, the one diagnosis that finally made the most sense to me—the one that explained the years of emotional landmines, relationship struggles, and inexplicable reactions to the world around me—was Complex Post-Traumatic Stress Disorder (c-PTSD).

Unlike standard PTSD, which is often linked to a single traumatic event, c-PTSD develops from prolonged exposure to repeated trauma—especially in childhood. It's what happens when the nervous system is trapped in survival mode for years on end, never fully shutting off the fight-or-flight response.

For me, c-PTSD wasn't just a diagnosis—it showed the early roadmap of my life. It's the reason my body tenses up at unexpected noises, why I sometimes struggle to remember entire chunks of my past, and why my emotions can go from zero to one hundred in a heartbeat.

And yet, strangely, this was the first label that didn't feel like an insult.

It framed my struggles not as personal failures, but as a *natural* response to *unnatural* circumstances. It wasn't a flaw in my personality, it was the result of a brain forced to adapt to a world that felt dangerous at every turn.

For the first time, I could look at myself and say, *I wasn't born this way. Life did this to me.*

But here's the real kicker: Trauma isn't just an emotional thief—it's a physiological vandal.

When Trauma Leaves Fingerprints on the Brain

Scientists have discovered that repeated trauma can actually alter the structure of the brain, particularly in regions like:

- **The hippocampus**, which controls memory and learning (so that explains the Swiss cheese effect on my recollection of events).

- **The amygdala**, which processes fear and emotional responses (cue my ability to overreact to the grocery store cashier's slightly condescending tone).

- **The prefrontal cortex**, which regulates decision-making and impulse control (hence my long-standing struggle with self-sabotage).

The effects don't stop there. Chronic trauma can also lead to immune system dysfunction, hormonal imbalances, and chronic inflammation—all of which I've dealt with in spades.

So, when people tell trauma survivors to "just move on" or "let the past go," I have to resist the urge to hand them a medical textbook. Because trauma isn't just something you remember—it's something your *entire body* carries.

Looking back, I can see how every single one of these psychological forces set the stage for my future breakdown.

Gaslighting taught me not to trust myself.

RSD made me desperate for approval.

CSA left scars that would take decades to face.

And **core-sounding** made sure that every negative experience built on the last, reinforcing the belief that I was inherently broken.

But here's the thing: trauma may shape you, but it doesn't define you.

And defining what broke me—and then what healed me—is precisely the mystery we're here to unravel.

CHAPTER 4: FROM INVISIBLE TO INVINCIBLE

In 1955, fresh out of high school and clutching my diploma with honors, I won a life-changing, two-month trip to Europe through a YMCA contest. It should have been a time of pure excitement—a golden opportunity to broaden my horizons and escape the suffocating familiarity of home. And yet, my thoughts weren't filled with dreams of grand adventures or romantic cobblestone streets. Instead, I was preoccupied with something far less glamorous: a boy who had zero interest in me. A boy who probably didn't even realize I existed.

Why did this bother me so much? Because I had just undergone what I like to call my "Cinderella transformation."

For most of my life, I had been a sickly, overlooked girl—my body bloated and tinged green from a failing kidney that had overstayed its welcome. When doctors finally removed the useless organ, my body flushed out years of built-up toxins, seemingly overnight. The puffy, sickly girl I had always been was gone. In her place stood a young woman who, much to my own astonishment, fit the 1950s beauty ideal with startling precision—slim, curvy, and, for the first time in my life, visible.

I leaned into it.

With this newfound confidence came a boldness I had never possessed before. I wrote six "Dear John" letters to various suitors, as if making up for lost time. I developed a knack for attracting men—something that had once seemed impossible. Let's be honest, the combination of a bubbly personality and ample cleavage didn't hurt in those days.

But even as my outward appearance shifted, the tangled mess of insecurities inside me remained. Therapy would later reveal that my fear of abandonment ran so deep that I had an unfortunate habit of sabotaging relationships before they had the chance to leave me first. Whether they were heading out in a submarine (which tragically sank) or moving back to England, I always made sure I was the one to slam the door before they had a chance to walk out. Classic defense mechanism.

Death by Balcony

Europe was supposed to be an adventure, and in many ways, it was—just not in the ways the YMCA might have approved of.

For one, I nearly sleepwalked off a balcony in England. Severe **somnambulism** (more commonly known as sleepwalking) had been a hallmark of my childhood, though, at the time, no one knew that such sleep disturbances could be an early sign of **Lewy body dementia.** Apparently, my unconscious self thought an impromptu second-floor dive was a great idea. Thankfully, someone caught me just in time.

That wasn't my only brush with trouble. There was also the police incident. Let's just say that while other students spent their prize money on cultural enrichment, I spent mine making memories that I can't quite repeat in polite company. What I *can* say is that I learned a valuable lesson: it's hard to appreciate fine European architecture when you're busy running for your life.

But despite all the chaos, my return home brought unexpected, good news. That fall, I was accepted into the Pasadena Playhouse of Performing Arts—a major achievement and, in my mind, the first real sign that my life was about to take a turn for the better.

A Star-Studded Start

Arriving at the Pasadena Playhouse felt like stepping into another world—one where raw talent, fierce ambition, and a healthy dose of off-stage theatrics reigned supreme. It was a sanctuary for dreamers, a proving ground for future stars, and, for me, a place where I finally felt like I belonged.

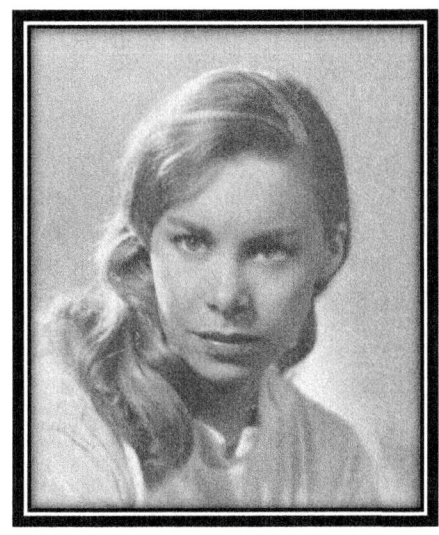

My Pasadena Playhouse Portrait

I threw myself into my studies with the kind of overzealous energy that only a young woman running from her own demons could muster. My grades were excellent, my acting was praised, and the dorm life wasn't half bad—though I did have a habit of stealing food from the common kitchen when the hunger pangs became too persistent.

But what truly made my time at the Playhouse unforgettable was the people. My roommate was none other than the Miss America runner-up. And my dorm mates? Well, let's just say they weren't exactly nobodies.

One of them was Ruth Buzzi, who would later become a comedic powerhouse on *Laugh-In.* Ruth was a force of nature—sharp, wickedly funny, and completely unforgettable. We performed together in *Dark of the Moon*, where

I had the lead role, but let's be honest—she stole the show as the head witch. That was Ruth. She could light up a stage like nobody else.

For the most part, this was a time of joy, discovery, and freedom. I adored my dance and theatrical makeup classes, but I also discovered another kind of attention that I wasn't quite used to—attention from boys. Oh, the boys!

One particularly persistent suitor was Kip King, a budding actor with undeniable charisma. Kip later became the father of *Saturday Night Live* comedian Chris Kattan, but back then, he was just a young man hopelessly in love with me. He even proposed.

And I declined.

To this day, I tease my children that if I had said yes, they might have ended up looking like Chris's hideous "Mango" character. Can you imagine? You're welcome, kids.

The Naïve Beard

Looking back at my twenty-something self, though, I hadn't yet given much thought to the fragility of identity or what it meant to lose oneself. If anything, I was still struggling to figure out *who* I was in the first place. At the Playhouse, I had mastered the art of becoming other people, slipping into roles with ease. But when it came to navigating real life, I was hopelessly out of my depth, stumbling through scenes without a script, uncertain of my cues.

Acting was second nature. Relationships? That was an entirely different performance—one where I hadn't quite figured out my lines.

During my first year at the Playhouse, I cautiously dipped a toe into the dating pool while stubbornly clinging to my virginity. My mother had warned me with utmost seriousness that *"sex will hurt unless you're married,"* and being the wide-eyed innocent that I was, I believed her wholeheartedly. It never even occurred to me to question the logistics of that statement.

Call it naïveté or deeply ingrained guilt—either way, I was fully convinced that the mechanics of it all somehow required a marriage license to function properly.

And then, there was the other part I didn't understand yet: I had a strange knack for attracting gay men.

Maybe it was my dramatic flair. Maybe it was my clueless charm. Whatever it was, I somehow found myself consistently cast in the role of the "beard" (a woman who dates or marries a gay man to provide cover for his homosexuality, a term I wouldn't learn until much later, when it suddenly explained an awful lot). I never questioned why these men weren't making any actual moves—I just assumed I was appealing enough to date, but not, you know, *that* appealing.

One of my more colorful suitors was Robert Eaton—tall, handsome, and dripping with mystery. He later became a well-known movie producer, married Lana Turner as her *sixth* husband, and got himself tangled up in a Howard Hughes book scam.

Naturally, when I heard about his infamous marriage, I rushed to grab Lana Turner's autobiography to see what she had to say about him.

She gave him exactly one dismissive paragraph.

Just enough to confirm that I wasn't the only one who had found him completely perplexing. Let's just say any lingering curiosity I had about him was firmly put to rest.

The Fencing Queen

While other girls at the Playhouse took up more traditional hobbies, I found myself drawn to something a little less conventional: fencing.

I was the only woman in the class, trained by the same fencing master who had once taught Errol Flynn—Hollywood's ultimate swashbuckler. I took to it surprisingly well, channeling my childhood trauma into every calculated thrust and parry. If I couldn't fight the demons in my head, at least I could stab them metaphorically with a foil.

It wasn't until years later that I learned traumatized people often feel most alive in the face of danger. It's part of the **fight-or-flight system**—our body's automatic response to perceived threats. And boy, did I lean into it.

Later in life, I'd find other ways to recreate that rush: dirt bike jumps, bareback horse riding at breakneck speeds, aggressive figure skating, and, let's be honest, an occasional bout of dangerous *invincibleness* (if that's even a word).

Looking back, it's no surprise I was drawn to the stage. Acting wasn't just about pretending to be someone else—it was a way to outrun the parts of myself I wasn't ready to face.

But as I was about to learn, no matter how far you run, you're *not* invisible—nor invincible—and life has a way of catching up with you.

CHAPTER 5: LUST, LOSS, & LEGENDS

While I was busy finding my footing at the Pasadena Playhouse, my beloved St. Bernard, Brandy, was finding his own claim to fame.

Brandy had been my loyal companion for years, a source of unconditional love in a world that often felt chaotic. But my stepfather had other ideas. Brandy's crime? Pooping in my sister's sandbox. That was all it took for him to be banished.

With no place for him at home and my hands full with school, I scrambled to find him a new home. The only option? Boarding him at a kennel while I worked at a movie theater to pay for it. But fate had a different plan.

Somehow—through sheer luck or maybe Brandy's natural charisma—he ended up in the care of Bob Hope's family. And not just as a pet. No, Brandy went on to a show-business career. My dog had officially outshined me in every way possible.

I was happy for him. Really, I was. But there was an undeniable pang of abandonment. It seemed even my own dog had moved on to bigger and better things without me.

Shoplifting for Sport

With Brandy gone and my anxiety at an all-time high, I found an unconventional coping mechanism: shoplifting.

Let me be clear—it wasn't about the thrill. I wasn't a kleptomaniac in the Hollywood-starlet-gone-rogue sense. It was about the odd sense of calm it gave me.

Department stores became my playground, and though I knew it was wrong, I justified my petty theft with the kind of logic only a traumatized mind could manufacture. After all, who's really hurt by a stolen lipstick or two? Answer: Nobody I cared about.

I never got caught, which only reinforced the habit. Psychoanalytic theory suggests that kleptomania is often linked to suppressing undesirable feelings or emotions. And in my case, it worked.

Decades later, after my return home from hospice, I found myself slipping into old habits—hiding things without explanation. Cookies, salt, tweezers. My son and his wife were baffled. Why was I doing this? I had no answer. Some things just become woven into your survival instincts.

Summer Stars and Scandal

The summer of 1956 was a whirlwind.

I landed a coveted scholarship to Rachel Rosenthal's acting studio in Los Angeles. Rachel, a legend in her own right, had trained at the iconic Actors Studio in New York. The experience was exhilarating.

Suddenly, I was rubbing elbows with Hollywood royalty.

I worked with Rachel doing improvisations alongside Tony Perkins, Natalie Wood, and Tab Hunter. Tab—Hollywood's golden boy—was as charming as he was stunning. During one acting exercise, which was set "at the beach," he stripped down to his underwear. Be still, my heart.

The world saw him as the ultimate all-American heartthrob. I, however, saw something more—a kind, unpretentious soul wrapped in a package of pure glamour.

But while my days were filled with acting, my nights were spent in a different world.

 I took a job at a coffee shop on Hollywood and Vine, serving an oddball mix of industry types and eccentric locals. Among the regulars? Vampira.

TV's original horror movie host, Vampira, would perch at the coffee bar in outfits so revealing they left little to the imagination—except for where she stashed her chihuahua, nestled snugly in her ample cleavage.

Between the shock factor of Hollywood nightlife and my own extreme immaturity, I wasn't prepared for the sheer chaos of it all.

By the end of the summer, I was shaken.

The things I had witnessed, the people I had met, the unsettling truths I had begun to grasp—it all felt like too much. So, I did what I always did when life overwhelmed me. I ran.

Back home, my parents took one look at me and dragged me to a psychiatrist. But the therapy sessions didn't last long. When the doctor hinted that my instability might have something to do with them, suddenly, my time was up.

Funny how that works.

Back to School, Back to Normal (Sort Of)

That fall, I enrolled at San Mateo Community College. For the first time in years, life felt stable.

I excelled academically and theatrically. I performed in plays, got good grades, and was even nominated for campus queen—though my fear of rejection kept me from participating in any of the hoopla around that.

My critical thinking professor once told me that I was his barometer for success. If my eyes lit up, he knew he had given a great lesson.

For the first time, I felt like I was on solid ground.

But, of course, trouble had my number on speed dial.

There was a fleeting crush on a younger co-star that made people whisper.

And then there was the Frenchman. Oh, that Frenchman.

His voice, which narrated my French language tapes, was so smooth and alluring that I practically melted every time I hit *play*.

I was a goner before he even said 'bonjour.'

Losing My Virginity: A Watermelon's Tale

At 20, I lost my virginity. Not in a romantic, candlelit moment. Not in a way that was sweet or special.

No, my deflowering came courtesy of a man named Jacques, a watermelon soaked in vodka, and a beach.

A few spiked slices later, I passed out in a sleeping bag. When I woke up, I knew.

Today, we would rightly call it rape.

At the time, in my naivety and shame, I saw that butchered fruit as a bitter metaphor for my own 'ruination.' I had lost the one thing I had fought so hard to protect.

And Jacques? He stayed in my life for a while. That's how deeply the web of learned helplessness and shame had trapped me.

Lust at First Sight

It was my second year at the Pasadena Playhouse when I saw him.

Tall. Dark-haired. Piercing green eyes. A jawline that could cut glass.

I turned to my friend and said:

"I'm going to marry that man."

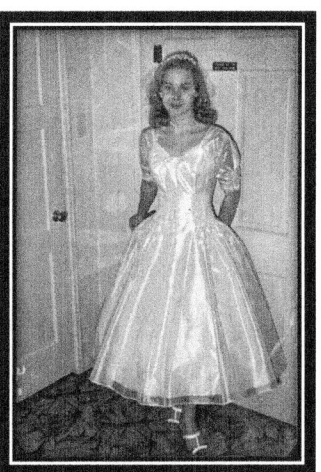

Three months later, I did, in a wedding dress I borrowed from my sister-in-law.

Jim Smith was everything I thought I wanted.

A small-town Korean War veteran from Colorado, he was charming, intelligent, and wildly attractive.

What I didn't know at the time was that he also came with a simmering alcohol problem.

But young love is the perfect blindfold for red flags.

Learning with the Legends—Dustin Hoffman & Gene Hackman

That same year, I had the privilege to play Dustin Hoffman's wife in two productions at the Pasadena Playhouse—*Danton's Death* and *As You Like It*. Sharing the stage with him was an experience like no other. Even then, he was intense, fully immersed in every role, dissecting characters with a kind of feverish obsession. His dedication wasn't just admirable, it was a little intoxicating.

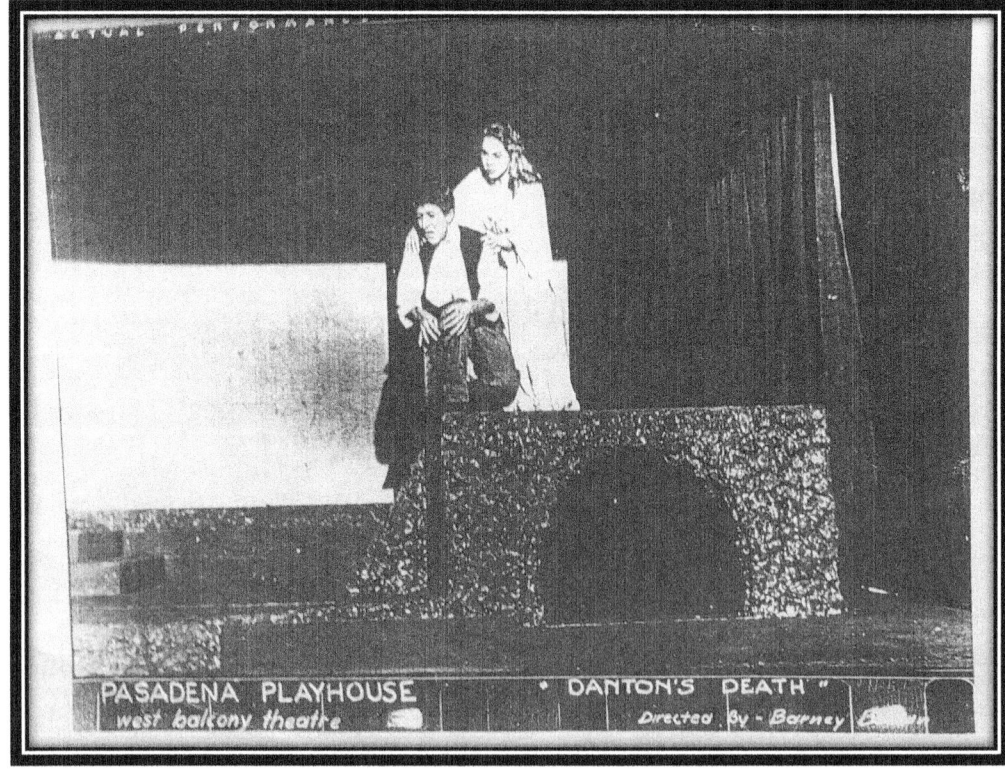

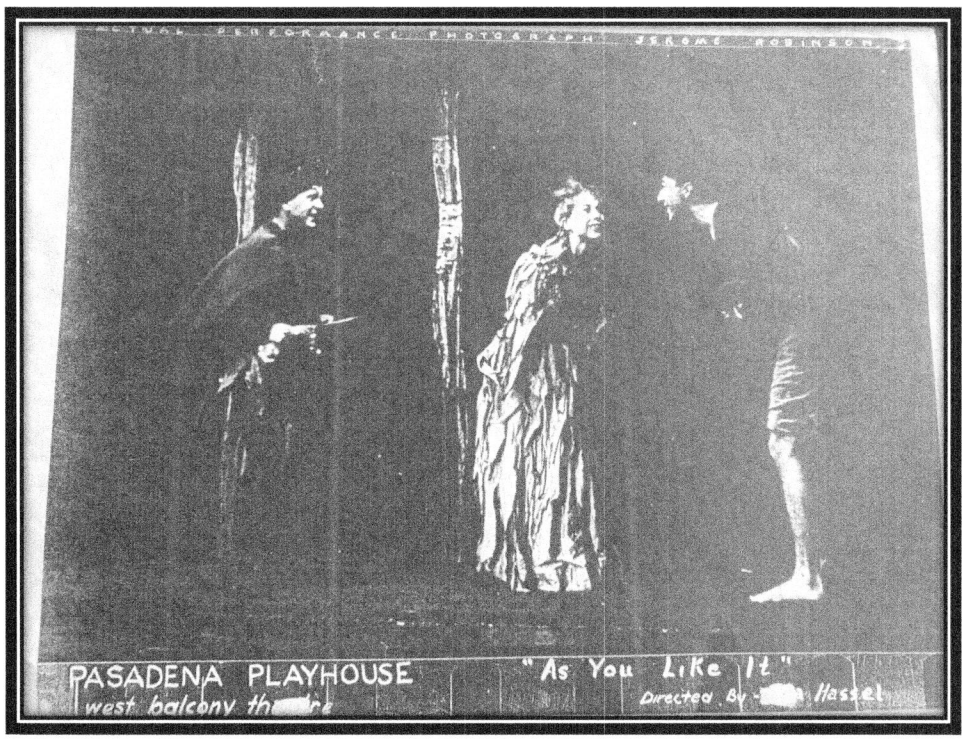

Dustin had a way of making everything about understanding people, especially women. He didn't just memorize lines; he studied emotions, reactions, body language. He wanted to know what made people tick. Years later, when I saw *Tootsie,* I laughed out loud. That was **him**. Every bit of it.

Once, in an effort to make our scenes "more authentic," he suggested we, well, "take things off, off-stage." He was charming and playful about it, but I turned him down. He took it in stride, never letting my rejection interfere with our friendship. If anything, it just made him more comfortable confiding in me about his various romantic entanglements. And trust me, there were plenty.

There came a time, like most struggling actors, when Dustin found himself unable to afford rent. So, he crashed with Jim and me in our tiny one-bedroom apartment. Space was tight, but Dustin, with his effortless charm, made himself right at home.

He had a self-deprecating wit that never faltered, like when he joked that his pants could stand up on their own because he never bothered to wash them. Classic Dustin—always fully committed to the role, even when there was absolutely no need for method acting.

Jim, my 6'4" cowboy husband, was amused by Dustin's energy. Dustin, in turn, gave Jim an affectionate nickname: "Matzo Balls." What inspired it, I'll never know, but Jim always took it as a compliment.

Everyone at the Playhouse knew that Dustin was bound for greatness. We laughed at his quirks, but always with admiration. His sheer brilliance made it obvious that his future was limitless.

Then there was Gene Hackman.

Gene was nothing like Dustin. Where Dustin filled a room the second he entered, Gene could disappear into the background. He wasn't withdrawn, exactly—just quiet, reserved, holding everything inside until it was time to unleash it on stage. He was like a coiled spring, storing all of his energy for the moment it mattered.

Dustin and Gene were thick as thieves, always pushing each other to be better. And hilariously, they had been voted "least likely to succeed" by our fellow classmates. Oh, the irony.

Unlike Dustin, I never acted alongside Gene, but we were in the same class, and you could *feel* his talent. He didn't perform so much as absorb his characters. It was as if he didn't have a personality of his own—he just *became* whoever he needed to be.

And now, **_he's gone_**.

The news of his passing hit me like a gut punch. Not just because we shared a classroom, a world, a time when we were all young, hungry, and reckless with ambition, but because of how cruelly his life ended.

Dementia didn't just take Gene Hackman—it erased him before he even left this world.

Reports say he didn't even know his wife of more than 30 years had passed away in the very same house. He was unable to call for help, unable to even feed himself, and a week later, he was gone too—most likely from starvation and cardiac complications (_Medical Examiner Reveals How Gene Hackman and His Wife Died_, 2025).

And what haunts me most is how preventable his suffering might have been.

Why wasn't he wearing a fall detection device? We live in a world where technology can track our every move, yet somehow, this man—this legend—was left alone in a house where no one knew he was dying. How does that happen?

For a man of his caliber, intelligence, and sheer presence to suffer such an ending is devastating. If only he'd been wearing a smartwatch, perhaps he could have been rescued.

I can't help but wonder: Did he ever feel afraid? Did he ever sense that something was wrong, that the world was slipping away from him piece by piece? Or was he, in some merciful way, too far gone to understand what was happening?

Dementia is a thief. It doesn't just steal memories—it steals dignity, identity, and everything that makes a person who they are.

The weight of Gene's decline lingers in my mind, stirring something deeper than just sadness—I am *angry*. Not at him, not at fate, but at the way society seems to view people with dementia, as though they've somehow ceased to matter the moment their memories begin to fade.

There's a stigma that comes with this condition, an unspoken belief that once someone reaches a certain level of decline, they are beyond help, beyond dignity, beyond worth. That they should simply be *thrown away*.

But that isn't true. A person's life doesn't suddenly lose all meaning just because their mind has been hijacked by an illness they have no control over. They may not remember us, but we remember them. And that has to count for something. Even in their diminished state, they are still *someone*—a life still worth honoring, a presence still worth cherishing.

Maybe they are no longer in control of their story, but that doesn't mean the story is over.

CHAPTER 6: DREAMS, DISASTERS, & DOMESTICITY

Jim and I were madly in love after graduating from the Pasadena Playhouse in 1958.

We had Hollywood dreams—big ones. Jim had the looks, the height, and the all-American charm that casting directors loved. While I dabbled as an exercise trainer, he went on audition after audition, hoping to land a breakout role.

One of his most promising opportunities was *Tarzan*.

It would have been a perfect fit—except for one problem. As a child, Jim had suffered from rickets, a disease caused by vitamin D deficiency that had left him with slightly bowed legs. And Hollywood, as it turns out, doesn't make loincloths for imperfect physiques.

That wasn't the only career roadblock.

Jim had landed a major role as Rock Hudson's brother in a big-budget film, and for a while, everything seemed to be falling into place. That is until Rock—Hollywood's reigning heartthrob—had him quietly booted from the movie.

At 6'4", Jim was taller, sharper, and, frankly, better-looking than Rock. But Hudson, every bit as beautiful as he was... let's just say, "not intellectually inclined," had no intention of sharing the screen with someone who might steal his spotlight.

Jim wasn't bitter about it, at least not outwardly. But between that and the *Tarzan* debacle, it became clear that Hollywood wasn't going to roll out the red carpet for us.

So, we pivoted.

We both auditioned for Desilu Productions, founded by Desi Arnaz and Lucille Ball, but neither of us got signed. It was then that I realized I was far too emotionally unstable to handle the brutal rejection of the industry.

So, I chose a more "stable" path—marriage and family.

Jim eventually gave up professional acting, too, though we found joy in community theater. Over the years, I poured my energy into plays, poetry readings, directing, decorating, and committee work at the Unitarian Universalist Church. No Oscars, but plenty of standing ovations from the church choir.

From Pasadena to a Mobile Home in Canada

It wasn't long before Jim and I packed up our lives and left California for the wilds of Eastern Canada to help his family.

His father had suffered a stroke, and their businesses were struggling. It wasn't exactly the glamorous Hollywood lifestyle we had imagined, but family was family, and Jim felt a duty to step in.

Our new home? A 35-foot single-wide mobile home parked on his father's property.

It was about as far from a fairy-tale start to marriage as one could get. But I tried to make the best of it.

My role in this adventure was secretarial—I handled correspondence for Jim's father's entertainment promotion business. And that's how I found myself writing a letter to Colonel Tom Parker, informing him that his young client, Elvis Presley, was scheduled for a performance in our town.

I never got a response.

Elvis never showed.

So much for my brush with rock 'n' roll royalty.

Still, I tried to find silver linings where I could. Jim's mother and I became close. She was a striking, accomplished woman, but also deeply bipolar. During one memorable Disneyland trip, she lost her dentures in a motel septic tank. Jim and his father spent hours fishing them out.

To this day, I have a vivid mental image of two grown men, sleeves rolled up, retrieving teeth from a foul-smelling abyss.

Marriage, it seemed, was full of unexpected moments like that.

Hairy Poodles and Hurricane Donna

In 1960, Jim and I packed up again—this time, heading for Jacksonville, Florida.

Jim had decided to study hotel management at Jacksonville University, and I took a job as a secretary. For a little while, life felt... almost normal. My mental state seemed to be on vacation, too, hanging out in the "abeyance" zone.

But Jim, ever the thrill-seeker, found ways to shake things up.

His latest hobby? Catching and releasing alligators for fun.

Yes, alligators.

Because what better way to unwind after a long day of studying than by wrangling prehistoric reptiles?

Not to be outdone by his own recklessness, Jim also shot a cottonmouth snake—a venomous, aggressive swamp monster—which promptly flew into the air and landed on his face.

I laughed until I realized I had married a man with a death wish.

While Jim was out tempting fate, I had my own moment of questionable bravery. At an amusement park, I decided to confront my lifelong fear of snakes and let a massive (but, thankfully, tame) serpent wrap itself around me.

Was it bravery? Was it stupidity? Who's to say?

Either way, I didn't die, and I even earned a little self-respect.

It felt like a metaphor for life in Florida: embrace the chaos, or let it eat you alive—literally.

Then came Hurricane Donna.

A Category 4 beast, Donna hit with relentless fury, flooding everything in sight. The water rose so high it nearly reached the floor of our trailer. At one point, a Coast Guard boat pulled up, ready to evacuate us to safety.

But there was a catch:

Our two shaggy standard poodles, Tinkerbell and Beau, weren't allowed in the shelter.

And we weren't about to abandon them.

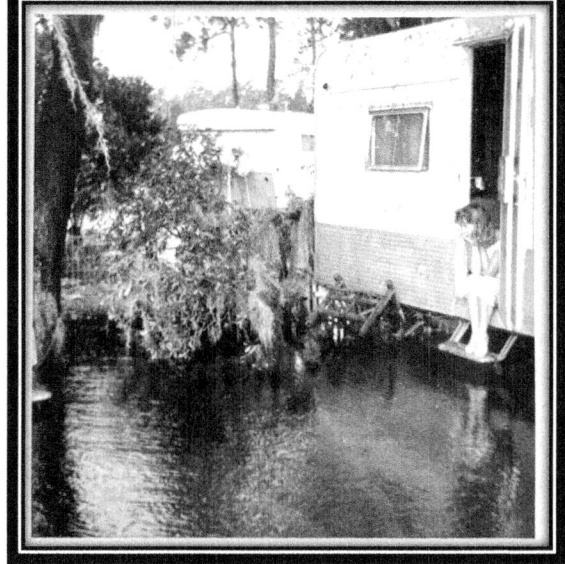

Viewing the flooding after Hurricane Donna

So, we stayed.

As we huddled inside, watching the storm rage around us, a heavy metal awning from a neighboring trailer flew past our window, missing us by inches.

It was five days of no electricity, no running water, and a whole lot of "Why didn't we think this through?"

Survival mode kicked in—well, for us, at least.

Tinkerbell, our spirited poodle, bit into an electrocuted fish that had latched onto an exposed wire.

Immediately, she went into a seizure.

We rushed her to the vet just in time to save her, but she was never quite the same after that.

Honestly? Neither were we.

A New Chapter and an Unthinkable Loss

Not long after, I found out I was pregnant.

For the first time in a long time, life felt full of light and possibility.

My pregnancy was blissfully normal—no complications, no warning signs. And yet, somehow, I never bought baby clothes. I never prepared a nursery.

It was as if a dark premonition lingered at the edges of my mind, unnoticed but present.

Then, the unthinkable happened.

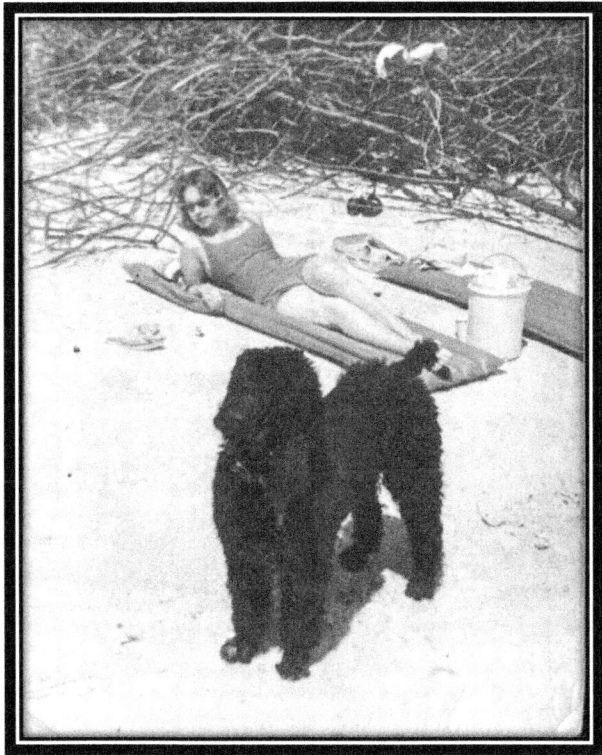

Newly pregnant on the beach with Beau

My baby girl was born with **osteogenesis imperfecta multiplex**, a rare genetic disorder that caused her bones to be as fragile as glass.

She passed away in my arms.

We named her Janet, in honor of the kind nurse who had cared for me during those devastating hours.

A tiny casket. A graveside farewell with just Jim and me.

No words can capture that kind of grief.

Grief in the Shadow of Joy

To make things even more unbearable, my sister-in-law—who lived in the trailer next door—had given birth to a healthy baby girl just weeks earlier.

Every time I saw her, every coo, every lullaby, every reminder of what I had lost, felt like a knife twisting in my heart.

Then, as if fate wanted to kick me while I was down, a simple trip to the grocery store ended with the cashier telling me that because my baby hadn't been baptized before she died, she'd be stuck in purgatory for eternity.

What does one even say to that?

Thank you for your unsolicited theology? Have a blessed day?

I walked out of that store feeling like I had been gutted all over again.

Jim and I were crumbling.

We had very few friends and no real support system in Jacksonville, no one to help us carry the weight of our loss. So, we did what people often do when the grief becomes unbearable—we ran.

Jim quit college. I left my job. We packed our belongings and left Florida behind, returning to California in search of something—*anything*—that felt like stability.

Soon, we were throwing ourselves into my family's wholesale business, The Sebrees, Inc. I told myself that if I just kept moving, if I stayed busy enough, I wouldn't have to feel the gaping hole in my chest.

CHAPTER 7: FRACTURED MINDS & FRAGILE BEGINNINGS

But grief doesn't work like that. It doesn't just pass through you—it settles in, rearranges things, and makes itself at home.

Back in California, I tried to return to some sense of normalcy. Besides working for The Sebrees, I also enrolled in a few classes and went through the motions of an "ordinary" life. But inside, nothing felt ordinary.

The panic attacks came first. Sudden, overwhelming waves of fear, each one accompanied by nausea, dizziness, and a crushing sense of doom. Then came the dissociation—those eerie, out-of-body moments where I felt like I was watching myself from a distance, detached from reality.

I knew something was wrong, something beyond just grief.

A psychiatrist confirmed my worst fears. After an evaluation, he diagnosed me with a "severe mental disorder"—one so serious, he warned, that it would require years of therapy.

Jim, however, wasn't having it.

His mother had been bipolar, her struggles laced with multiple suicide attempts, and he couldn't bear the idea of having a "mentally unbalanced" wife. Therapy was a luxury he wasn't willing to entertain, and just like that, any chance of professional help was gone.

So, I did what I had always done—I endured.

I buried the panic attacks, the dissociation, and the depression and carried on, forcing myself to appear normal. But inside, I was barely holding it together.

Hope Reborn: Ty and Shawn

Then, a miracle happened.

I became pregnant again.

For nine months, I was a nervous wreck. Every twinge, every flutter, every second without movement sent me into a spiral of worst-case scenarios. I had lost one child—what if I lost another?

But this time, the universe was kinder.

Ty was born healthy, pink, and full of life, and in that moment, my world shifted. It was as if the universe had cracked open just enough to let the light back in.

Two years later, Shawn arrived, equally perfect in my eyes.

While **postpartum depression** (a condition causing mood swings, anxiety, and fatigue after childbirth) occasionally crept in, motherhood became my anchor, the thing that kept me from drifting too far into the abyss. I poured myself into it completely—sewing matching outfits for the family, planning zoo trips, remodeling our little house in an upscale neighborhood.

I was determined to give them a childhood free of chaos, fear, and instability. But life, as always, had other plans.

Ty: The Brilliant Hurricane

Ty wasn't like other children.

Even as a toddler, there was something different about him—something that set him apart in ways I couldn't quite articulate. He was reading novels at six, skipping grades, and charming strangers with his piercing eyes and impossible intelligence.

But he was also exhausting.

At one prestigious nursery school, Ty made history—not as the brightest student (which he absolutely was) but as the first and only child to require a leash. His hyperactivity was off the charts, an endless whirlwind of movement and ideas that no one, not even me, could keep up with.

The specialists confirmed what I had already suspected: ADHD, predominantly hyperactive-impulsive type.

The doctors suggested Ritalin, the go-to medication at the time. We gave it a shot, desperate for a reprieve from his boundless energy. But instead of calming him, it backfired. The "rebound effect" hit him hard, making him more wired, more erratic, and more uncontrollable than before.

So, we stopped.

Instead, we got creative.

Physical affection wasn't exactly Ty's thing—he hated hugs with a passion. So, Jim and I developed a game. We'd sit on the floor, pretending to "scare" him into hugging us. It worked, sort of, and provided plenty of laughs along the way.

Years later, when *The Big Bang Theory* debuted on television, I immediately recognized him.

"Sheldon Cooper is Ty," I told my family.

They all agreed. Ty was Sheldon—right down to the literal interpretations, social missteps, and overwhelming intelligence.

Shawn: The Gentle Fighter

Shawn's entrance into the world wasn't as smooth as his brother's.

During delivery, the umbilical cord wrapped tightly around Shawn's neck, cutting off his oxygen supply. In a matter of seconds, his tiny body turned blue, motionless. Panic surged through the room, but Jim didn't hesitate—he sprinted down the hall, desperate to find more help. By some miracle, they got to him just in time, resuscitating him before it was too late.

We never told Shawn the full story. He knew about the cord, of course, but not about how close he had come to never taking his first breath, nor the potential effects it might have had on his life. We thought we were protecting him, sparing him from carrying the weight of a "what if" that couldn't be changed. But now, looking back, I wonder—was it really the right choice?

Shawn was the opposite of his brother in almost every way—quiet, gentle, and content to live in the background while Ty stole the spotlight. He was the textbook example of a "glass child"—a term for siblings of those with disabilities, children who are often overlooked because their parents' energy is consumed elsewhere.

But even in his quiet nature, Shawn was remarkable.

His kindness, his resilience, his ability to weather the chaos of our family without resentment or bitterness—it was something truly special.

As the years passed, life was not always kind to him. His adult years were marked by hardship, and recently, he suffered a small stroke.

For three long years, we lost touch. My own battle with dementia, my time spent in senior care facilities, my return home—it all blurred together. But then, one day, Shawn surprised me with a visit.

Seeing his face again after so much time was like medicine to my soul.

We talked. We healed.

Having him back in my life, even if just for a while, reminded me that love has a way of finding its way home.

The Stepford Illusion

On the surface, life looked perfect.

I was the ideal 1960s housewife—frilly aprons, homemade meals, doting mother, loving wife. But underneath the polished exterior, my mind was unraveling.

The panic attacks returned, accompanied by bouts of **agoraphobia** (fear of being in situations where escape might be difficult) and episodes eerily similar to what I would later recognize as early symptoms of Lewy body dementia.

There was no trigger, no warning. Just a sudden, all-consuming sense of impending doom.

And then, one day, I ran away.

Not permanently. Not in any grand, dramatic way.

I just... left.

I checked myself into a YMCA for women, desperate for air, space, something—anything—to quiet the noise inside my head. But it didn't last. Jim found me, brought me home, and life resumed its usual rhythm.

We made a decision then: two kids were enough.

Jim scheduled a vasectomy.

We arrived at the appointment, settled into the waiting room, and prepared for what was supposed to be a routine procedure. But just as the doctor was about to begin, he collapsed in front of us, seizing violently—a full-blown grand mal seizure taking over his body.

And just like that, the surgery was off the table—at least for the moment. In an instant, fate had stepped in and temporarily saved the family jewels.

Jim, ever the tough guy, wasn't fazed. We promptly found another urologist, and when he did eventually have the procedure done, he simply hopped on his Harley and rode home as if riding a motorcycle post-surgery was just another Tuesday.

The House That Broke Me

Around that time, we decided to renovate a house, dreaming of turning it into a beautiful showplace.

It was a disaster.

An architectural magazine called it "a thorn among the roses," which was a polite way of saying, "What were you thinking?"

I was humiliated.

The criticism sent me into a spiral of self-doubt and depression so deep that I could barely function. For a month, I wallowed, questioning every decision I had ever made.

Eventually, we moved to Fremont, determined to start fresh.

This time, I got it right.

I transformed the interior of that house into a tasteful sanctuary and turned the landscaping into a true design triumph. This time, no critics—magazine or otherwise—were invited to weigh in.

It wasn't flashy, but it was cozy, stable, and, most importantly, devoid of any resemblance to past design disasters. For the first time, it felt like we had a true family nest—no thorns in sight.

But it wasn't just about the house, it was about rebuilding myself.

Balancing on the Tightrope of Life

Jim was a loving father, but life didn't exactly deal us an easy hand. It threw curveballs like a major league pitcher on a winning streak, and we were constantly adjusting, dodging, and sometimes getting hit square in the face. Between navigating Ty's brilliant but challenging mind and guiding Shawn through his quieter, more tender struggles, we did our best—with plenty of mistakes and more than a few exasperated sighs along the way.

Through hurricanes, heartbreaks, and a series of surreal and often absurd moments, we survived. Looking back, I don't just see the chaos, I see the resilience we built, sometimes unknowingly.

My mental health felt like a high-wire act without a safety net, always teetering on the edge. Life was unpredictable, often messy, and frequently ridiculous, but somehow, I kept moving forward, even when the music stopped playing.

And then, for a fleeting moment, life granted me something unexpected: a pause.

CHAPTER 8: SOLITUDE & SELF-DISCOVERY

The summer of 1968 should have been a brief oasis in the chaos of motherhood—a chance to rediscover myself without the constant chorus of "Mom! Mom! MOM!" echoing through my days. Jim packed up the boys—then four and six—and took them to Canada to work with his father, leaving me alone for the first time since giving birth.

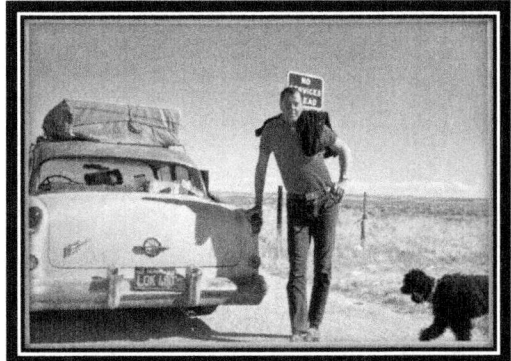

I had big plans for this time, imagining I'd find my inner peace and maybe even develop a sophisticated new hobby like painting or French cooking. Instead, I moved back into my mother's house, took a job as a clerk, and promptly got fired for insubordination—because, apparently, I wasn't great at following rules. (A shock to absolutely no one.)

Jim heading to Canada with the boys

Determined not to waste this rare moment of independence, I enrolled in medical secretarial classes, which I genuinely enjoyed. But let's be honest—San Francisco was still buzzing with the aftershocks of the "Summer of Love," and I wasn't about to spend all my time buried in textbooks.

I'd love to tell you that I spent my free time expanding my mind with philosophical discussions and deep existential reflections, but in reality? I was mostly just soaking in the joy of having zero responsibilities. The freedom was—if you'll excuse the pun—*intoxicating.*

And yet, even in those blissful moments, there was always a small voice in the back of my mind whispering, *"This won't last forever."*

Because, of course, it didn't.

The Return to Reality

Like a cruel alarm clock jolting me awake, Jim and the boys came back, and just like that, my brief taste of independence was over. But this time, something felt different. We settled into a rhythm that actually seemed...stable.

I landed a job as an administrative assistant to the chief of staff at Kaiser, a position I adored. It felt like the first real step toward a career, something I could be proud of.

For a brief moment, everything was falling into place.

And then, in true fashion, life decided to throw a wrench into the works.

Ty's Brush with Death

Ty was seven years old, which meant he was essentially a tiny stuntman with no sense of self-preservation.

One day, his impulsive streak got the best of him. He darted into the street without looking—and right into the path of an oncoming car.

I don't remember thinking. One second, I was standing there, and the next, I was sprinting toward my child, his tiny body crumpled on the pavement, blood spreading beneath him.

His foot had been badly gashed open, bleeding profusely. Panic took a backseat to instinct. I grabbed him, flagged down the closest driver, and screamed, "TAKE US TO KAISER!"

Somehow, we made it there in time. One of the best orthopedic surgeons in the world—who also happened to be the 49ers' team doctor—operated on him. Later, he even testified in the trial against the drunk driver who hit Ty.

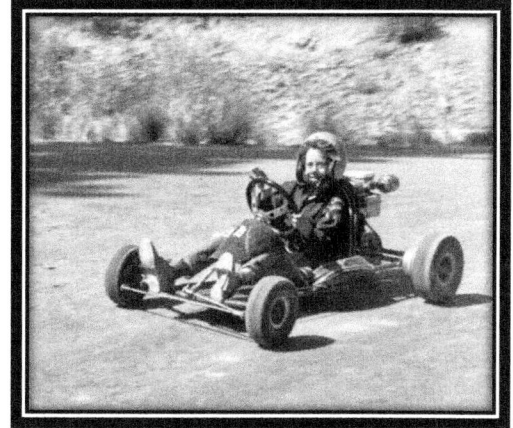

Ty's foot healed, though it was never quite the same. But in true Ty fashion, he refused to let it slow him down. He went on to run cross-country in high school, proving that resilience ran just as strong in his veins as recklessness.

Jim, ever the pragmatic problem-solver, built Ty a go-kart so he could join us on dirt bike rides while he recovered. If he couldn't run just yet, at least he could race.

The Making of a Daredevil

Ty's accident should have instilled caution in me. Instead, it seemed to ignite something even wilder.

I threw myself into adrenaline-fueled escapades, embracing my new title as the daredevil mother.

Dirt bike trail jumping became my escape—soaring through the air, landing (mostly) without injury, and racking up ER visits like a frequent flyer program.

The nurses at Kaiser knew me by name, and I wore my scrapes and bruises like trophies.

Ty, always watching, absorbed my recklessness like a sponge. I knew it wouldn't be long before he'd be right beside me, chasing the same thrill.

The Simmering Battle with Alcohol

For years, I had been adamantly against drinking. My father's battle with alcoholism had been a living cautionary tale, and I swore I would never follow the same path.

And yet...

Jim had always struggled with drinking, and for a long time, I tried to curtail it, going as far as watering down his whiskey bottles in secret.

But eventually, I caved.

At first, it was just social drinking—a glass here, a sip there. But before I knew it, alcohol had become a coping mechanism.

I wasn't drinking for fun anymore.

I was drinking to manage stress.

I was drinking to numb emotions I didn't want to deal with.

I was drinking to keep up with Jim.

And soon, opioids entered the picture—although I never obtained them illegally, they were prescribed and always justified. But addiction isn't about legality; it's about dependence.

Addiction—what's now called **Substance Use Disorder** (a chronic, relapsing brain disorder characterized by compulsive drug seeking, continued use despite harmful consequences, and long-lasting changes to the brain)—isn't a moral failing. It's a disease that changes the brain's wiring, making it harder to quit. Studies show that oxytocin (a hormone involved in social bonding) can reduce the effects of alcohol on the brain's reward center, though it didn't seem to help me much.

I had slipped into a dangerous cycle, and I wasn't sure how to climb back out.

The Life-Altering Accident on the San Mateo Bridge

Jim's drinking might have continued unchecked if not for his near-fatal car crash on the San Mateo Bridge.

One night, while crossing the bridge, Jim collided with a stalled garbage truck, its lights conveniently failing at just the wrong time. The impact knocked him unconscious, leaving him bleeding and broken in the wreckage.

And then, in a moment that could have been ripped straight from a bizarrely scripted redemption arc, the Hells Angels appeared.

Yes, the Hells Angels.

What a twist of fate this was: Sonny Barger, the notorious longtime president of the Hells Angels motorcycle club, and a few of his gang just happened to be nearby. Spotting the mangled car, they sprang into action, pulling Jim from the wreckage and stabilizing him until help arrived. As they loaded him into the ambulance, Jim briefly regained consciousness. Sonny leaned in and, with a grin that could almost make you forget his reputation, said, "We're not all bad guys."

Jim's injuries were severe—he required surgery for an aortic dissection (a life-threatening tear in the artery wall). The operation was performed by the legendary Dr. Norman Shumway, a pioneering heart surgeon renowned for performing the first human-to-human heart transplant.

You would think cheating death would be the wake-up call Jim needed.

It wasn't.

Instead, Jim spun a tale so convincing that I actually believed it.

He told me the surgery had been "only *partially* successful," and that the best possible treatment was whiskey.

Yes. Whiskey.

Naive as I was, I believed him, never questioning why the world's top heart surgeon might prescribe bourbon instead of beta blockers.

That was the moment I should have woken up.

That was the moment I should have stopped making excuses.

That was the moment I should have walked away.

But I didn't.

Instead, I let it continue, let it unravel everything until the damage was too great to ignore.

And the worst part?

I was right there, spiraling down with him.

CHAPTER 9: DONKEY BASEBALL & DESPERATION

By the time Jim left the family business, his drinking had spiraled entirely out of control, and our lives became a chaotic mess of one lost job after another, financial ruin, and half-baked survival strategies. We had already gone from homeowners to serial renters, each new place more humiliating than the last. At one point, we even had to pawn my mother's wedding ring just to make ends meet, and if you're wondering—no, I never saw that ring again.

If there was one unexpected silver lining in all of this, it was that my kids always found ways to keep life interesting—even in the middle of our financial and emotional meltdown.

Take the time Shawn nearly bit his tongue in half.

I don't even remember the exact details of how he managed to do it, but suddenly, there was blood everywhere and an ER visit waiting to happen.

Ty, being the opportunistic little schemer that he was, saw an untapped business venture in his brother's misfortune.

With Shawn's badly swollen, grotesquely infected tongue on full display, Ty marched him around the neighborhood, charging curious spectators for the privilege of gawking at the carnage.

Yes, my son turned his brother's medical emergency into a money-making sideshow.

And people paid.

I suppose I should have been horrified, but honestly? At that point in my life, I respected the hustle.

Another Great Escape

During this turbulent period, I clung to any semblance of normalcy, trying to keep my world from completely unraveling. One of my more questionable strategies was sticking close to my Uncle Glen and his family, hoping that being around familiar faces might stabilize things.

That plan imploded rather quickly.

Something happened—though to this day, I still don't know exactly what.

Either my sister seduced their youngest son, or I made some wildly inappropriate comment in one of my classic, unfiltered defense mechanisms (a skill I have honed over decades, often to my own detriment).

This might also explain why I love *The Far Side* online forum so much—it's one of the few places I can say whatever I'm thinking without having to apologize for it later.

But even that awkward disaster pales in comparison to what came next.

Jim's mother, who had struggled for years with severe bipolar disorder, took her own life using sleeping pills.

We were already barely holding things together, but this? This was the final straw.

Jim wasn't making any ends meet selling used cars, and I was too emotionally drained to keep pretending we weren't drowning.

It was clear that we needed a drastic change—and what's more drastic than moving to a 100-acre farm in Ontario, Canada, where Jim's father had now started a... well, let's call it a "unique" business venture?

That's how we found ourselves trading California instability for Canadian absurdity, stepping into the wild, wild world of Donkey Baseball.

When the Family Business Involves Hooved Chaos

For the uninitiated, Donkey Baseball is exactly what it sounds like: a regular baseball game—except that every player but the pitcher, catcher, and batter, has to ride a donkey.

And if you think donkeys are cooperative animals, you have clearly never met a donkey.

Some refused to move, no matter how much coaxing was involved. Others took off running at the worst possible moments. A few were known for aggressive bucking, launching unsuspecting riders into the air like rag dolls.

The announcers had a field day with it, tossing out quips like, "There goes Preacher Jones on his ass."

Yes, people actually paid money to watch this spectacle.

And in case you're wondering, Donkey Baseball was a legitimate thing back then—an actual touring event that was just as ridiculous as it sounds. We weren't the only ones cashing in on the absurdity, but we certainly had our share of "memorable" moments.

Becoming a Donkey Whisperer

Since we were fully committed to this strange new life, I decided I would take on the role of self-appointed donkey trainer.

The donkeys had distinct personalities, and it didn't take long to figure out which ones would gently trot along, which ones would pretend to comply before launching their rider into the dirt, and which ones would stand still like statues until the game was over.

And then there were the baby donkeys—the absolute sweetest creatures on earth. Within minutes of being born, they would teeter around on wobbly little legs, playing hide-and-seek in the tall grass, their soft muzzles practically begging for endless petting.

It was impossible not to fall completely in love with them.

But despite my affection for the babies, I quickly learned that managing a donkey business wasn't all laughter and fuzzy moments.

Every spring, the male donkeys had to be gelded—because if left intact, they would enthusiastically mount each other with what I'll politely refer to as "great vigor and highly visible equipment."

It wasn't exactly something we could ignore—unless we wanted to turn every community Donkey Baseball event into an R-rated fiasco.

So, guess whose job it was to ensure the whole process went smoothly? That's right—yours truly.

Springtime meant following around the freshly castrated donkeys with a bottle of fly spray, making sure their healing wounds didn't attract swarms of opportunistic insects.

Probably the worst job ever.

I sometimes wondered if this was karmic retribution for something I'd done in a past life—because surely, somewhere, some ancient ancestor of mine was laughing hysterically at my predicament.

Creating a Viral Sensation (Before That Was a Thing)

One of the most infamous moments in our family's Donkey Baseball history happened when our kids' school hosted a game as a fundraiser.

Ty, ever the mischievous trickster, suggested that his school principal should ride one of our more "spirited" donkeys.

The principal, being a good sport, agreed.

So, naturally, Ty chose Silver, the most aggressive, unpredictable donkey in the entire herd.

And Silver did not disappoint.

Within seconds of mounting, the principal was bucked into the dirt in front of a delighted audience of children and parents.

The kids were howling with laughter. The principal? Less amused.

But in that moment, I reveled in the glow of cool-mom status, feeling like a true hero in their eyes.

A Birthday Party for the Ages

But it wasn't all fly spray and questionable life choices; there were genuinely joyful moments, too.

That year, 1969, Ty and Shawn's joint birthday party turned out to be one of my favorite memories (they turned eight and six, respectively).

Naturally, given our current donkey-centric lifestyle, the theme of the party had to be donkey-related.

The kids played a hilariously modified version of *Pin the Tail on the Donkey*, using tape instead of pins for very obvious reasons (because, let's be honest, the last thing I needed was a lawsuit over an accidental donkey stabbing).

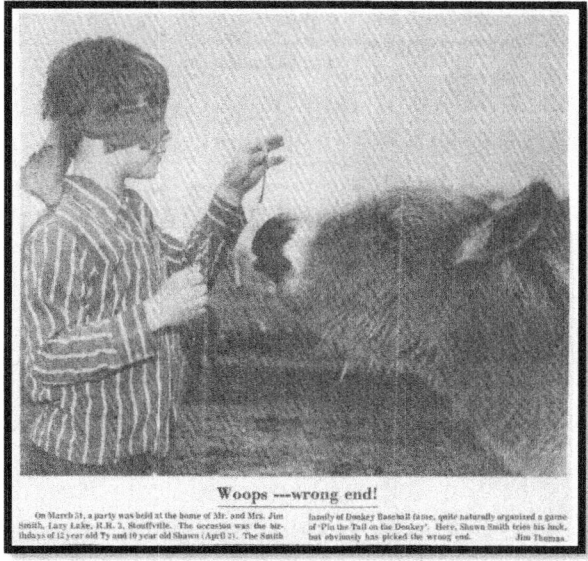

Woops ---wrong end!

On March 31, a party was held at the home of Mr. and Mrs. Jim Smith, Lazy Lake, R.R. 3, Stouffville. The occasion was the birthdays of 12 year old Ty and 10 year old Shawn (April 2). The Smith family of Donkey Baseball fame, quite naturally organized a game of 'Pin the Tail on the Donkey'. Here, Shawn Smith tries his luck, but obviously has picked the wrong end. — Jim Thomas.

But the real highlight was Shawn, in all his adorable enthusiasm, proudly sticking the paper tail directly onto the donkey's nose instead of its rear.

The sight was so endearing and ridiculous that a local newspaper featured a picture of it, capturing a moment of pure, unfiltered childhood joy.

CHAPTER 10: A BEAUTIFUL, BIZARRE LIFE

Moving to Ontario, Canada, had been like stepping into a dream—a sprawling 100-acre property overlooking the lake, with rolling green pastures, towering trees, and a serenity that seemed almost surreal.

It was supposed to be a fresh start—a geographic escape from Jim's spiraling alcoholism and our crumbling financial situation in California. I collaborated with an architect to design the perfect Tudor-style cottage overlooking the lake, and together, we brought it to life. For a time, it truly felt like our own little slice of heaven.

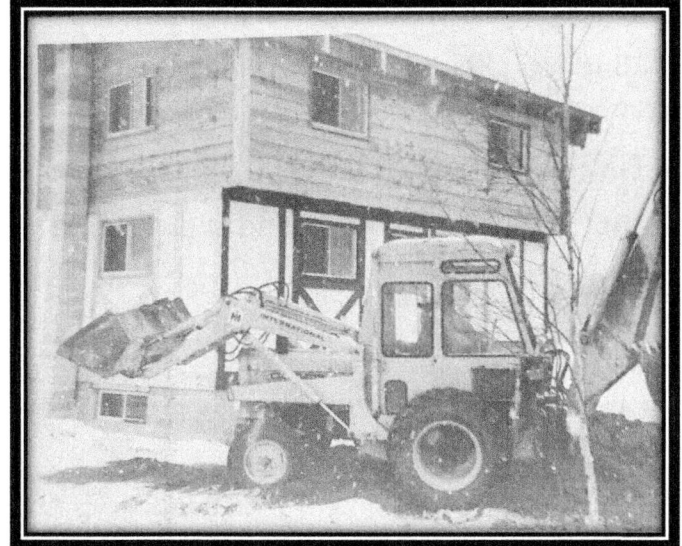

Jim's father had funded this new beginning by purchasing the property with a chunk of my inheritance (which, in hindsight, was perhaps not my best financial decision, but I was operating on blind optimism at the time).

At first, the land felt like a sanctuary—a place where we could breathe, where the kids could run free, and where Jim and I could rebuild our marriage.

Except it didn't quite work out that way.

A Family Circus in the Worst Way

Life in Ontario was idyllic on the surface, but underneath, it was a tangled mess of family dysfunction and questionable life choices.

The main source of chaos was Jim's new stepmother—a woman so unhinged and volatile she could have inspired an entire season of a true crime documentary.

She had recently lost her previous husband, who—get this—threw himself in front of a subway train after discovering her affair with Jim's dad.

Rather than, say, taking some time to reflect on her choices, she had moved on with Jim's father at lightning speed and was now running our household with all the grace of a rabid raccoon in a locked pantry.

She had borderline personality disorder—every day was a new emotional rollercoaster—and I was just another passenger trapped in the front row.

As if that wasn't enough family drama, I was also drinking more than I cared to admit.

I told myself it was just to keep up with Jim, but deep down, I knew I was self-medicating—desperately trying to drown out the noise of my own unraveling reality.

And then, as if the universe decided I needed one final humiliation, there was the furniture polish incident—which, let's just say, taught me a very valuable lesson about what does NOT make a good substitute for alcohol.

Venus the Horse: My Saving Grace

Just when I thought I might actually lose my mind, Jim surprised me with a gift that would change everything—a gorgeous palomino horse named Venus.

Venus was part Clydesdale, which meant she was a force of nature— muscular, steady, and built for endurance. She carried herself with a quiet strength, the kind that made you believe in second chances, in something solid and dependable when the rest of the world felt anything but.

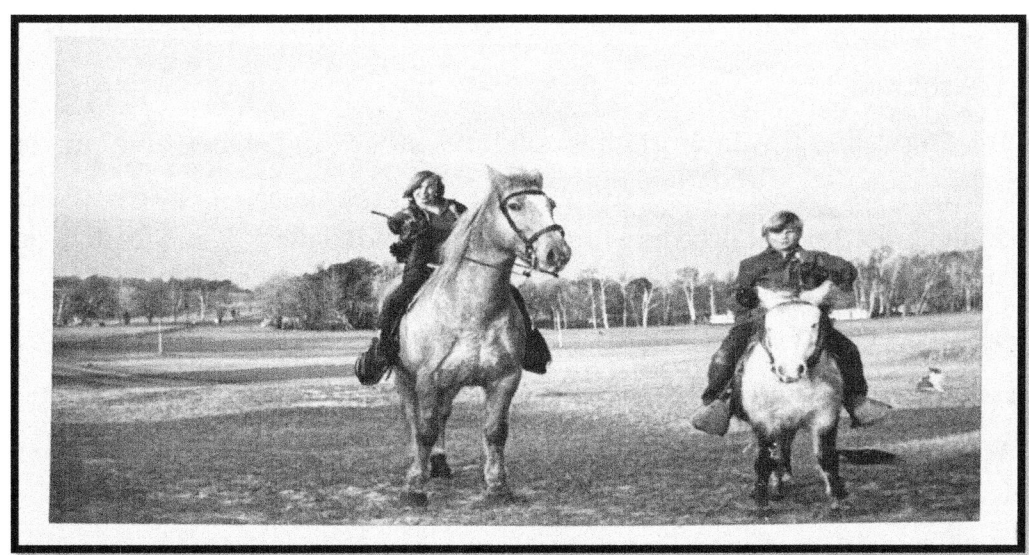

Ty on Venus & Shawn riding Dolly

She quickly became more than just a horse—she was my refuge, my escape, my steady companion when life was shaking me to my core. With the boys riding alongside me—Ty on Lynn, his standard-bred pony, and Shawn on Dolly, his sturdy Highland pony—we explored the vast Canadian wilderness for hours.

The rhythm of hooves against the earth, the sheer openness of the land—it was the closest I had felt to freedom in ages.

I even joined cattle drives, which sounds a lot more glamorous than it actually was. Turns out, herding cows is less like a Western movie and more like an exhausting battle of wills.

Still, I loved every second of it.

Venus and I also dabbled in show tricks—if I shifted my weight just right, she would paw at the ground on command, and I proudly told anyone watching that she was "counting."

The locals were impressed, though I suspect Venus was just humoring me, playing along with my little charade.

Still, I couldn't help but think she would've fit right in back at the Pasadena Playhouse—graceful, commanding, and always ready to steal the show.

Horsing Around with Logistical Challenges

At some point, we decided that Venus should have a foal—a logical next step, right?

Except for one minor issue: she was massive, standing at almost 18 hands tall, which made finding a suitably sized stallion an interesting challenge.

The solution?

Digging a literal trench for her to stand in so the smaller stallion could "reach."

Sadly, our efforts at breeding failed, but that didn't stop Venus from making unauthorized visits to the stallion's farm every chance she got.

Clearly, she had her own plans, and I had to respect her determination.

Seasons of Joy and Survival

Winters in Ontario were bone-chillingly brutal, but they brought a whole new level of adventure.

We hitched Venus to a sled and tore through the snow, laughing until our faces were numb.

Come springtime, I had to shave the "feathers" off her legs to make her look more refined—a task that probably took longer than any human haircut I've ever given.

And summer?

That was when Venus and I swam together in the lake—her powerful body moving effortlessly through the water while I clung to her like some kind of half-drowned rodeo queen.

Those were the moments I held onto—the ones that made me believe that, despite everything, there was still beauty to be found in the chaos.

A New Purpose: Helping Others

As much as I loved life with Venus, there was one thing missing—a sense of purpose beyond survival.

So, in 1971, I took a job at Participation House, working with severely disabled children, and, for the first time in a long while, I felt truly fulfilled.

I had always felt a connection to individuals with disabilities—maybe because, in many ways, their resilience mirrored my own struggles.

One particularly joyful summer, we invited the children and their families to our property for a picnic.

Watching them laugh, ride Venus, and experience pure happiness was one of the greatest moments of my life.

For one beautiful afternoon, there was no dysfunction, no trauma—just joy.

And that was enough to keep me going.

What a Paradox

But life in Ontario was a paradox—both a sanctuary and a slow-motion disaster, filled with breathtaking beauty, unpredictable chaos, and unexpected moments of peace.

Between family madness, a drinking problem I wasn't ready to confront, and a horse that somehow understood me better than most humans ever did, it was a chapter in my life that shaped me in ways I never could have predicted.

Looking back, I see it for what it really was:

A season of survival.

A lesson in resilience.

But what I didn't yet realize—a big storm was coming, and I had no idea just how hard it would hit.

CHAPTER 11: A HARD RESET

I wanted Ontario to be the fresh start we needed.

I wanted to believe that Jim's drinking would stop, that our family could rebuild and that we could find stability in our sprawling Canadian paradise.

But reality had other plans.

That job at Participation House may have fed my soul, but it certainly didn't feed the family. Jim's alcoholism had only worsened, and with harsh winters, money troubles, and dysfunction creeping into every corner of our lives, we had to face the truth—it was time for a separation.

Not a divorce, at least not yet, but enough space for him to attempt sobriety in rehab while I tried to hold things together for the kids.

Leaving Ontario meant leaving behind Venus, the breathtaking landscape, and the home and life we had painstakingly built.

But it also meant leaving behind the chaos that was swallowing us whole.

And so, in 1975, with Ty and Shawn in tow, I boarded a plane back to California, carrying only a suitcase of essentials and a heart weighed down by uncertainty.

Returning to the Past, But Not as the Same Person

Back in San Carlos, we moved into my mother's sprawling home, a place that, while familiar, felt nothing like home anymore.

I took a clerk job back at The Sebrees, Inc., always hoping that Jim would send for us after getting the help he needed.

The successful, thriving wholesale business my parents owned was now, unfortunately, on its last legs.

The current economic downturn was just the beginning of these hard times. The retail landscape was also shifting, with big-box stores like Target and department stores crushing the small gift shops we supplied.

To make matters worse, my conniving stepbrother had already jumped ship, taking our best customers with him to start a competing business.

Oh, and let's not forget my stepfather's declining mental state, a brutal combination of brain cancer and dementia, which meant his increasingly violent outbursts were just another cherry on this collapsing sundae.

Everything was falling apart.

So, like I always did, I tried to fix it.

Parenting in Crisis: The Kids vs. Chaos

By 1977, Jim had finished his stint in rehab, so the boys began spending their summers back up in Canada with him—right in the heart of the Donkey Baseball circus. While Jim managed the spectacle of grown men attempting to play baseball atop stubborn, uncooperative donkeys, my boys found their own ways to stir up mischief and create a different kind of chaos.

Come fall, after returning to school in California, Ty quickly proved himself a prodigy—not just in long-distance running, but also in the art of skipping textbooks altogether. He was one of those rare individuals who could coast through school on sheer intellect, seemingly absorbing knowledge through osmosis while the rest of us had to put in actual effort. But raw intelligence doesn't always come packaged with sound decision-making, and at seventeen, he was arrested for speeding.

When I got the call, I had a choice: rush to bail him out or let him spend the night in jail. My gut told me to leave him there—not as a punishment, but as a lesson.

Now, before you slap a "Worst Mother of the Year" sticker on my forehead, let me add this: at the time, I was literally working part-time for the police department, counseling people on how to navigate the justice system. So, there I was, sitting across from worried parents, giving them advice on how to get their kids out of jail while mine was locked up just a few cells away.

But Ty, being Ty, somehow managed to turn jail into a redemption arc. While other kids might have panicked, he spent the night comforting and protecting a mentally challenged boy who was being bullied by other inmates. When I finally picked him up the next day, the officers actually praised him. Leave it to my kid to walk into a jail cell and come out looking like a hero.

Then there was Shawn—the social butterfly, the charmer, the master of skipping school. Getting him to class was like trying to convince a cat to take a bath. In one of my more misguided attempts to ensure his attendance, I let one of Ty's friends drive him to school in Ty's brand-new car—a car he had just recently purchased with the funds from his accident settlement.

You can probably guess what happened next.

The friend wrecked it. To this day, the memory of that decision makes me cringe.

In the midst of all this, I found myself so overwhelmed that, in a moment of sheer desperation, I actually called the Children's Abuse Prevention hotline for parenting advice. Imagine being so lost that you willingly call a number designed for actual abuse cases just to figure out how to survive raising teenagers.

But let's be honest—there is no manual for this. Just a series of gut punches, facepalms, and the occasional glass of wine (or three).

The Business That Refused to Be Saved

By 1982, after my mother and stepfather had both retired, I threw myself into reviving The Sebrees, determined to breathe new life into what was left. My sister even joined the company as a salesperson and worked incredibly hard to keep us out of the red.

I redesigned the inventory, created new marketing strategies, and managed to increase revenues again with my innovative buying skills. Riding that sales wave gave me the courage to put together a catalog that I thought would revolutionize our approach and really add a 'wow factor' for our customers.

It was artistic.

It was clever.

It was a total disaster.

Customers hated it.

Sales plummeted, and I had to swallow my pride along with a generous helping of self-loathing.

That's when it hit me:

I wasn't meant for this kind of work.

I didn't care about selling products—I wanted to *help people*, to create something meaningful, to work toward something that actually mattered.

And yet, here I was, stuck in a failing family business, trapped by obligation and dwindling options.

But it wasn't just the business that was doomed—it was my sense of direction.

Hoping to Live Long & Prosper

For years now, there had been one form of relaxation that gave me more solace than I might care to admit—watching reruns of *Star Trek* and, dare I say it, being somewhat of a "Trekkie."

Ty and I watched religiously, drawn to its vision of a future where humanity had finally gotten its act together. A world where people had overcome their worst instincts—a future of peace, equality, and boundless discovery.

I didn't just watch *Star Trek*; I absorbed it. I went to conventions, actively participated in the fandom, and became an engaged member of the fan club. We weren't just entertained by it—we studied it. Its themes, its lessons, its blueprint for a world where people actually treated each other with dignity.

But the irony is that I had unknowingly contributed to *Star Trek's* legacy before I even realized it.

Years earlier, while living in Thousand Oaks, I attended a Unitarian Universalist (UU) fellowship—one that just so happened to count *Star Trek* creator Gene Roddenberry as a fellow member. One of the first *Star Trek* writers, Jerry Sohl (also a UU member), had even consulted *me* while developing the show's first episode. In one of our conversations, I suggested that the series should integrate UU principles into its foundation—values like human dignity, justice, and exploration.

Knowing that my input—however small—was woven into the fabric of *Star Trek* filled me with a quiet, undeniable pride.

It was one of the few things in my life that hadn't turned to ashes.

The Shadows in the Background

Yet, even with our newfound obsession, I couldn't ignore the storm clouds still hanging over us.

Shawn's downward spiral hadn't stopped.

Ty, despite his brilliance, was struggling socially.

And me? I was barely keeping it together, clinging to whatever scraps of hope I could find.

The move back to California had given us distance from the worst of the chaos, but I knew it was only a temporary fix.

I was running out of time, running out of ideas, and running out of energy.

Something had to change. And soon.

A New Home and a World of Wonder

Eventually, the tension of trying to revive that failing business and my stepfather's dementia-filled rages—fueled by a cruel cocktail of brain cancer and Alzheimer's—in our home became unbearable.

So, I packed up the boys and moved into a tiny apartment, determined to create a new life for us.

It was during this time that Ty's fascination with *Star Trek* deepened, and I found myself fully immersed in it alongside him.

For Ty, *Star Trek* wasn't just entertainment; it was a roadmap for the kind of world he wished existed.

For me, it was a temporary reprieve from a reality that had offered me nothing but disappointment and loss.

And in a way, it gave me hope—if not for myself, then for the next generation.

Maybe Ty, with his brilliant mind and unwavering belief in a better world, would be one of the people who actually helped make it happen.

I just needed to make sure he had the chance to try.

Looking Back: A Hard Reset

One day, as I stood in our tiny, quiet apartment, I realized something:

Returning to California was supposed to be a reset, but it felt more like a slow-motion disaster.

I had lost my husband to alcohol, my business to circumstance, my sense of purpose to failure, and my peace of mind to the relentless chaos of it all.

And yet, I had survived more than most people ever would.

Was I broken?

Sure. But I wasn't done yet.

As I looked at Ty, buried in another *Star Trek* episode, and Shawn, whose path was still uncertain, I realized something:

This chapter of my life wasn't an ending. It was a hard reset.

And the next one?

It was going to test me in ways I couldn't yet imagine.

CHAPTER 12: FROM BLACKOUTS TO BREAKTHROUGHS

By the early 80s, self-improvement wasn't just a trend—it was practically a religion, and I was ready to worship at the altar of personal enlightenment. After all, I had survived a failing business, financial ruin, and the emotional whiplash of single motherhood. Surely, the key to fixing my life was out there. And so, like a moth to a flame—or, more accurately, a stressed-out single mom to a pseudoscientific fix-all—I found myself sitting in a packed seminar room, staring down the latest guru promising transformation: Erhard Seminars Training, or EST.

It was two weekends of psychological boot camp, a 200-person crash course in breaking down your psyche through sheer exhaustion. The rules were simple: no food, no sleep, and no bathroom breaks for hours on end. We were told it was all part of the process—discomfort breeds enlightenment—but what I mostly felt was hunger, exhaustion, and an overwhelming urge to punch someone in the face.

The entire ordeal culminated in a grand crescendo where participants were expected to leap to their feet and proclaim, "I've gotten it!" as though some cosmic truth had been downloaded directly into their souls. I, however, remained firmly planted in my seat, arms crossed. What had I "gotten"? A headache? A newfound distrust of groupthink? A creeping realization that I had just spent a small fortune to be held hostage in a room full of sleep-deprived zealots?

EST was just the tip of the iceberg. Sensitivity training, encounter groups, and every self-help fad you can imagine were sweeping the country, turning personal growth into an extreme sport. I became a regular at these so-called "growth centers," chasing the promise of emotional healing. What I found instead was coercion, manipulation, and what could only be described as psychological dodgeball.

In one particularly twisted exercise, I was forced to scream my darkest confessions into the face of a near-stranger—who, as fate would have it, was a man whose advances I had politely declined in real life. Now, under the guise of "therapy," he had full permission to hurl insults, accusations, and whatever repressed anger he had stored up. The leaders, drunk on their own power, encouraged these confrontations, some even crossing the line into physical aggression.

These sessions were emotional war zones, and the casualties were real. The worst part? I willingly signed up for them, convinced they held the answers to my suffering. I guess when you're desperate for healing, you'll believe just about anything.

The Home That Wasn't

There's a moment when you realize that everything you built, everything you fought for, is crumbling beneath you. For me, that moment stretched into years.

By the mid-80s, The Sebrees, our family business, was circling the drain, and I was desperately still trying to keep it afloat. My mother, who had sacrificed so much to keep it going, was devastated. My sister, who depended on her paycheck, suddenly had nothing. And my kids? Let's just say my track record as a mother at that point wouldn't win me any awards.

With nowhere else to go, I moved into the company warehouse. A tiny camping trailer became my home, with a small wooden room built for Ty in the warehouse (Shawn had already struck out on his own). There was no running water. No kitchen. My hygiene routine consisted of sneaking into the warehouse bathroom and heating water in a Mr. Coffee machine. I told myself this was temporary; that I could turn things around.

But the truth was, I was unraveling faster than an old sweater caught on a nail.

The Last, Worst Decision

One night, drowning in box wine and despair, I decided I was done.

No more clawing my way through the mess I had made. No more pretending. No more failing.

I taped up the windows and doors of my trailer, turned on the gas, and waited for oblivion.

But because the universe has a dark sense of humor, the butane ran out before I did.

I woke up the next morning to a pounding headache and the cold, inescapable truth: I had *failed* at failing.

At the time, it wasn't funny. Now? I've learned to laugh at the absurdity of it all. That moment—ridiculous as it seems in hindsight—was the lowest I had ever been.

And yet, somehow, I still had further to fall.

Hope from Venus

Amid the chaos, Jim—of all people—sent me Venus, my beloved horse, all the way from Canada. She was a constant, a thread of peace I could still hold onto. Riding her through the mountains of California gave me fleeting moments of clarity. Once, we even encountered a mountain lion, and Venus calmly guided us to safety, unshaken by the danger.

She was everything I wished I could be—graceful, fearless, steady.

But horses are expensive, and I could barely keep myself alive, let alone a 1,200-pound animal. With a broken heart, I gave her to the family of a little girl who adored her, saddle and all. I could have sold everything for thousands of dollars, but her happiness meant more to me than money.

It was one of the hardest things I had ever done. And it pushed me even deeper into the void.

Spiraling into Madness

If my life up to that point had been a series of bad decisions, what came next was the grand finale of self-destruction.

At some point, I made the brilliant decision to take one of my dog's tranquilizers—which, at the time, was a variant of LSD—before another dreaded dental appointment.

But instead of a less stressful visit with the dentist, I had a full-blown meltdown in a McDonald's on my way there. I was so off the rails that the staff called the police. I managed to escape before they arrived, but if I ever needed proof that my life had utterly derailed, that was it.

And then, Jim threw me one last curveball—divorce papers. Turns out, he had moved on with a nurse he met at an addiction clinic. At least one of us was getting better.

Ty and Shawn had already flown the coop, leaving me alone with my mess. So, in true dramatic fashion, I packed up my things and ran straight into the arms of George Johnson, my former Unitarian Universalist minister.

A Love Affair with an Expiration Date

But George wasn't just *any* minister. He was a poet, a recording artist, and a civil rights activist who had marched with Martin Luther King in Selma. And

I was... a hot mess in a flowing muslin dress, drifting through life like a lost extra from a Woodstock documentary.

We had a whirlwind, passionate affair. But reality hit fast. I was a free-spirited flower child. He was a respected man of God. Our worlds weren't just different, they were incompatible.

Eventually, I did what made the most sense for both of us: I left. George didn't take it well. He called, drunk and pleading, begging me to come back. But I ignored him. Partly because I was done, and partly because there's only so much poetry-spouting, whiskey-fueled begging a girl can take.

Vanish and Start Over

It didn't take much longer before The Sebrees met its inevitable demise. A perfect storm made from the increasing popularity of big-box stores, my stepbrother's shady dealings, and my own addiction-fueled incompetence took it down for good.

When the end came, I pulled a Houdini.

I abandoned the warehouse entirely—left behind all the goods, the trailer, the office equipment—everything. For a brief stint, I even lived in my car.

(Pro tip: A car makes a terrible studio apartment. And the trunk? Not as spacious as you'd think.)

After stringing together some secretarial temp jobs, I managed to scrape together enough money to move into a tiny studio apartment.

But, like most things in my life at the time, it didn't last.

Laurel House: A Second Chance at Survival

The night Shawn found me in a suicidal blackout was the night everything changed. (I'm not sure of the details because it's still a complete blur to me.)

He pulled me from the abyss and took me to rehab. That's how I ended up at Laurel House, a live-in recovery program where I spent nine months rebuilding my life.

The housemother and counselors gave me something I hadn't had in years: structure. Stability. A reason to keep going.

For the first time in what felt like forever, hope flickered.

From Garbage Bags to New Beginnings

When I left Laurel House, everything I owned fit into a single garbage bag.

No suitcase. No money. No place to call home.

During my time in rehab, Josh moved into my old studio apartment, but returning there was never an option. The memories were too raw, too suffocating. So, everything I had—furniture, belongings, pieces of my past—was simply left behind.

Instead, I moved in with a fellow recovering addict. That didn't last, either. She relapsed, and I had to pack up and move on... again.

Leaving Rock Bottom Behind

Survival isn't guaranteed.

Not everyone makes it.

I learned that the hard way.

After nine months at Laurel House, the bonds I had formed with other women in recovery felt unbreakable. We had fought together, cried together, and rebuilt ourselves together. But in the real world, without the structure and safety net of rehab, too many of them slipped back into the darkness.

We tried to stay connected, meeting in coffee shops and recovery circles, clinging to each other like survivors of a shipwreck. But one by one, they fell. Some convinced themselves they could drink in moderation. "Controlled drinking," they called it. I knew it was a lie, but that didn't stop me from testing the theory myself later on.

I failed. Spectacularly.

And for some, the failure was fatal.

There was one friend in particular; brilliant, funny, and deeply wounded. She called me—completely drunk—on my first day working at Suicide Prevention. I listened, but I had to cut the conversation short when my boss came over because we weren't supposed to handle calls from family or friends.

That night, she stepped in front of a truck.

She was gone.

And the weight of her loss still lingers.

Throwing Myself into Recovery (And Side-Eyeing AA)

Her death shook me to my core. I didn't want to end up like her.

So, I did what I had always done when faced with disaster: I doubled down.

I threw myself into recovery with the same obsessive determination I had once given to self-destruction.

I went to 100 AA meetings in 100 days. I played the game. I became a sponsor.

But some things about AA never sat right with me. The idea of *powerlessness*, for one. I had spent my entire life being powerless. The thought of surrendering even more control didn't feel like salvation—it felt like more of the same.

And then there were the "thirteenth steppers."

Older men, circling like vultures, preying on vulnerable young women just trying to rebuild their lives.

I saw it happening to my own sponsee. I watched these men exploit recovery like it was their personal dating pool.

It made me sick.

That's when I started exploring other programs. I found <u>LifeRing</u> and <u>Women for Sobriety</u>, which focused on self-empowerment and accountability.

They resonated with me in a way that AA never did.

For the first time, I wasn't just surviving. I was *rebuilding*.

Blacking Out & Breaking Through

Of course, life after rehab wasn't all smooth sailing.

In fact, it was just as bizarre, humiliating, and surreal as everything that had come before.

Take, for example, my job working the hotline at Suicide Prevention (which eventually morphed into the Director of Volunteers).

Not only was I working there, I was about to read my own file.

Not many people get the once-in-a-lifetime opportunity to flip through a detailed archive of their lowest moments.

But there it was. A giant, mortifying stack of documented evidence.

I had made so many blackout calls for help that the volunteers had actually started recognizing my voice—even when I used fake names.

I thought I had been clever. But yikes, I sure wasn't.

Then I found it—the final entry.

A slurred, desperate plea I had no memory of making.

It stared back at me like a bad punchline to a long, painful joke.

And for the first time, I truly saw myself.

No more excuses. No more pretending.

I **had** hit rock bottom. And I had the paperwork to prove it.

Rebuilding, One Strange Job at a Time

With no money, no bank account, and nothing but a garbage bag full of belongings, I did what I had to do:

I worked.

First, I cleaned my psychologist's house in exchange for therapy sessions. Glamorous? No. Necessary? Absolutely.

Then came the weirdest job of all—working for a minister who sold Osborne computers (one of the first "portable" computers, if by "portable" you mean lugging around something the size of a sewing machine).

Instead of a paycheck, he paid me in computers.

I had zero use for them, so I handed them off to my boys, who were thrilled. Finally, something good came out of my employment history.

But the minister had a side hustle, too.

Deprogramming cult victims (and writing bestselling books about it, no less).

And when he was too busy, I filled in.

Yes, you read that correctly—I, a recovering alcoholic with a wildly unstable life, was now assisting in cult deprogramming.

It was exactly as disturbing as it sounds.

His methods? Somewhere between psychological warfare and a full-scale intervention with no exit strategy.

I lasted just long enough to lose all faith in humanity.

I quit before I needed to be deprogrammed myself.

From Chaos to College

Meanwhile, back at home, my newest roommate had descended into full-blown, raging alcoholism.

I needed *out*. Fast.

At an Overeaters Anonymous meeting, I overheard a woman saying she had a room available—but only for college students.

So, naturally, I enrolled in San Mateo Community College (SMCC) the very next day.

Desperate? Maybe. Resourceful? Absolutely.

That decision changed everything.

My Unexpected Career Path

One career-planning class was all it took.

That's where I discovered speech-language pathology.

It was a perfect blend of everything I loved—medicine, theater, instruction, empathy.

It felt like I had spent my entire life accidentally preparing for this career.

From blackout calls to working towards a master's degree—it wasn't the easiest path, but it was mine.

For the first time in forever, I had direction.

I wasn't just moving forward.

I was building something real.

CHAPTER 13: WHEN ONE DOOR CLOSES

They say that when one door closes, another opens.

But what they don't tell you is that sometimes, you have to kick that damn door down yourself, armed with nothing but sheer determination and a questionable sense of humor.

So that's exactly what I did.

Newly divorced, the boys grown and off living their own lives, I decided it was time to do something for myself. Time to stop surviving and start *building* something real.

I went back to college—thanks, in large part, to the VA, which helped cover the cost as a benefit from my father's WWII military service.

And somehow—against all odds, against every chaotic twist in my life—I earned my Master of Science in speech-language pathology.

Math: My Arch-Nemesis

Of course, getting to that degree wasn't without its hurdles.

Because of all my severe kidney issues in high school, I had missed months of classes and barely attended part-time after my surgery. Back then, homeschooling wasn't an option, and my math education? Well...let's just say it never happened.

Algebra? Never heard of her.

So, when I had to take placement tests to qualify for university-level classes, the results came back grim. I was mathematically frozen in time—stuck at a *sixth-grade level*.

Yes. Sixth grade.

I hadn't felt that humiliated since I had to parade my uniform in front of the headmistress for "outgrowing" it.

But I refused to let numbers get the best of me.

Armed with nothing but a self-study workbook and sheer stubbornness, I threw myself into a remedial math class at SMCC. And I didn't just *pass*. By the end of the semester, I was acing college-level algebra, logic, and statistics like I had been born to crunch numbers.

That year flew by, and soon, I transferred to San Francisco State University—where, coincidentally, Ty was also enrolled, pursuing a career in journalism.

Coffee Breaks and Life Lessons

We would often meet for mother-son coffee dates, and I would jokingly tell my professors that if they dared give me a bad grade, Ty would *"expose"* them in the school paper.

Watching him thrive filled me with pride.

Meanwhile, Shawn was working at a laundry, married, and busy expanding the family with three adorable boys. Babysitting my grandsons and taking them on little adventures became one of my greatest joys.

Through it all, I stayed fiercely devoted to my recovery.

I attended LifeRing and Women for Sobriety group meetings religiously, soaking up every bit of wisdom they had to offer. Kaiser's dual-diagnosis rehab meetings (for addiction and bipolar disorder) became another crucial part of my foundation.

By the time 1988 rolled around, I had something to show for all my hard work: my undergraduate degree in speech, language, and hearing.

It was a moment of triumph. The first step toward an entirely new chapter.

Balancing Family Life and Earthquakes

My college years weren't *all* academic achievements and personal growth.

Sometimes, they were pure adrenaline.

Take 1989, for example.

There I was, sitting in graduate school, enduring an impossibly dull child education class, doing everything in my power to stay awake—when *BOOM*.

The floor rolled. The walls *shuddered*.

The infamous 7.0 San Francisco earthquake had struck.

While everyone else dutifully followed safety protocols and was herded toward the stadium for "protection," I had *other* plans.

Ignoring every official directive, I bolted to the parking structure, determined to rescue my car and race home to check on my family.

Five stories of concrete above me? Didn't care.

Potential aftershocks? Didn't care.

All that mattered was getting to my car, getting on the road, and making sure everyone was okay.

Luckily, my family was fine. My little rented cottage in Palo Alto sustained some damage, but nothing I couldn't handle.

My cat, however, never forgave the earthquake.

The chair she had been sitting in when the earth decided to rearrange itself became permanently *cursed*. She refused to sit there ever again.

Honestly? I couldn't blame her.

Because if there was one thing I had learned by that point, it was that life had a way of shaking things up—sometimes literally.

A Visit from the Past

A few weeks after the earthquake, my ex-husband, Jim Smith, came back to California for a family visit. Time had done its work—his once jet-black hair had softened into a distinguished silver, but the charm was still intact. So was the drinking.

When we met, he wasted no time trying to convince me that we should pick up where we left off—marriage, intimacy, the whole package. I would be lying if I said I wasn't tempted. He was, after all, Jim—ruggedly handsome, effortlessly charismatic, the man I had once loved. But I had worked too hard for my sobriety, too hard for my education, and I wasn't about to let nostalgia (or loneliness) derail me.

So, with a bittersweet heart, I said no.

Still, we stayed in touch, talking regularly over the phone, our history too deep to fully let go. Five years later, he passed away from heart disease and Parkinson's in a Canadian skilled nursing facility. Shawn attended his funeral. I wasn't there, but I mourned him just the same.

Typing My Way into a Career (and a Little Trouble)

Somewhere between my graduate studies and keeping my life afloat, I decided I needed a better job. Kaiser was hiring medical transcriptionists, and though I had zero experience, I had two things going for me: solid anatomy grades and lightning-fast typing skills.

During my interview, they administered a typing test. Halfway through, the buzzer went off as the interviewer took a call. Thinking quickly, I did what any resourceful (or mildly desperate) student would do—I kept typing. When they asked if I had stopped at the bell, I smiled sweetly and said, *"Of course."*

That little fib got me the job.

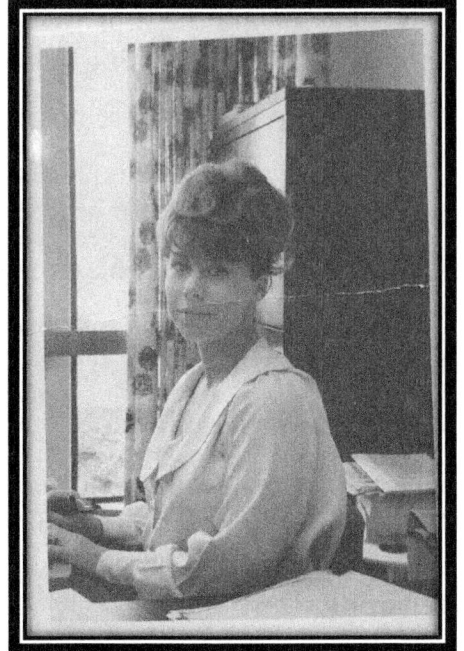

Of course, the problem with bluffing your way in is that you eventually have to prove you belong. It didn't take long for my boss to realize that while I was a fast typist, I was a clueless one. But instead of firing me outright, she handed me test tapes and told me to practice after hours.

I practiced, all right. Just... not on the test tapes.

Instead, I quietly polished the *real* dictated reports—admissions, operative notes, radiology findings—turning them from raw, error-filled transcripts into professional, publish-worthy documents. My boss never caught on, but soon, my "practice" paid off. I wasn't just surviving, I was excelling. Before long, I went from a fumbling newbie to a full-time employee.

It was my own personal "Kobayashi Maru" moment—bending the rules like Captain Kirk, beating the system.

Years later, when I returned to Kaiser as a speech-language pathologist (SLP), those same transcriptionists—who had once watched me fake my way through the job—greeted me with applause and congratulations. Now, *I* was the one dictating reports. That full-circle moment felt like a victory lap with a side of poetic justice.

Straight A's, a Full-Time Job, and Premonitions

Balancing work and school was like juggling flaming torches while riding a unicycle—but somehow, I pulled it off.

I worked full-time as a medical transcriptionist, took *up to 21 units* a semester (which required special permission because, apparently, the university assumed students needed things like "sleep" and "sanity"), and still managed straight As.

Financially, I scraped by on academic aid, scholarships I tracked down like a bounty hunter, and side hustles—cleaning houses, temping, whatever it took to keep going.

Then, one day, as I was drowning in textbooks and stress, I thought to myself, "If I could just injure myself enough to take time off work, I could really focus on studying."

The universe, as always, was listening.

Not long after, I tripped on the stairs and broke my arm. Just like that, I had my wish—occupational disability leave. Careful what you wish for, indeed.

This wasn't my first eerie brush with premonitions. Over the years, I'd had more than a few moments where life seemed to *whisper* its plans before they unfolded.

Like the time I casually predicted my healthy grandmother would pass soon—and she did.

Or when I refused to buy a single baby item during my first pregnancy, despite having no reason to expect complications—only to tragically lose the baby at birth.

I can't explain it. It's not something I try to make sense of. It's like my brain occasionally gets sneak previews of life's plot twists, whether I want them or not.

Maybe it's intuition. Maybe it's just terrible timing. Either way, I've learned to pay attention.

Academic Triumphs

Premonitions aside, I graduated *early* and with high honors. At the ceremony, I stood as the English Department's designee, my name listed under more scholarships than any other graduate. It was a moment of triumph, a tangible reminder of how far I had come.

But the true highlight came when my son, Ty, repositioned my class ring. It was such a simple gesture, but it carried the weight of everything I had fought for—every long night, every struggle, every moment I had doubted myself.

On top of my master's degree, I also earned my Certificate of Clinical Competence (CCC), which required an additional year of coursework, a clinical practicum, and a postgraduate clinical fellowship. No one tells you that becoming a speech-language pathologist feels like leveling up in a particularly grueling video game, but trust me—it does.

From Cutting Throats to Fetching Condiments

It didn't take long before I secured a highly competitive fellowship at the San Francisco VA Hospital. Under the mentorship of an incredible supervisor, I dove headfirst into the deep end of medical speech-language pathology.

One of my first major challenges was creating a laryngectomy social group—bringing together patients who had undergone total laryngectomies to help them adjust to life without vocal cords.

The other challenge? My supervisor thought I was ready to place a Blom-Singer indwelling voice prosthesis—a process that involved cutting through the skin of a patient's neck to expose the trachea and performing tracheoesophageal punctures—an advanced procedure not typically done by SLPs. It was a terrifying, high-stakes task, especially for a newly minted clinician. My first patient was incredibly stoic, which was fortunate because my protective mask kept fogging up from sheer panic.

When my fellowship ended, I landed my first official job as an SLP at an upscale skilled nursing facility in Palo Alto. My very first solo patient?

Someone from my past.

She had been at Laurel House when I was there for live-in alcohol rehab, and let's just say she wasn't exactly my biggest fan.

But life, as it often does, has a way of rewriting our stories.

A stroke had left her with severe **dysphagia**—the swallowing dysfunction that would later become my specialty. I treated her, she recovered, and despite our history, she was grateful.

Not every job was so poetic, though.

My next gig was at a senior day program, where I arrived in my best "professional SLP" attire, eager to begin my work—only to be handed a tray and told to serve lunch.

Between tying bibs and refilling drinks, I checked the swallowing function of the residents. It wasn't glamorous, but it was real, and the motivated seniors I worked with quickly won me over.

The Whiteout Incident

Eventually, I set my sights back on Kaiser, hoping to return—this time, as an SLP.

During the application process, they requested a simple medical report. Any recent doctor's visit would do, they assured me.

Easy enough.

Until I saw what the report contained.

Right there, in black and white, was a full account of my addiction history and the medications I had taken for my mental health.

I knew how the world worked.

No matter how qualified I was, no matter how much I had rebuilt my life, the stigma of addiction and mental illness could be enough to sink my chances before I even got through the door.

So, I did what I had to do.

I grabbed my trusty bottle of whiteout, carefully erased the damning details, and submitted a clean copy.

Was it ethical? Probably not.

Did it work?

Absolutely. I got the job.

CHAPTER 14: USING WHAT LIFE (AND DEATH) TAUGHT ME

Redwood City Kaiser was a neurological center, a place where I felt like I had stumbled into the perfect intersection of learning and purpose. I wasn't just working, I was absorbing, refining, and sharpening my skills. And the specialty that captivated me most? Dysphagia.

At the time, I had no idea just how personal that would become.

While I was busy learning how to diagnose and treat swallowing disorders, my stepfather—someone who had inflicted his fair share of pain on me and my sister—was living out his final days in a skilled nursing facility. His dementia, brought on by brain cancer, had stolen his mind. But it wasn't the cancer or the dementia that ultimately killed him.

It was aspiration pneumonia.

A complication of dysphagia.

The very thing I was training to prevent.

I don't know if I would call it irony, fate, or some cruel joke from the universe, but the weight of it stayed with me. No matter how complicated my feelings toward him were, I couldn't ignore the fact that his death—avoidable, preventable—was the same kind of tragedy I would spend my career fighting against.

And so, I turned that weight into action.

The "Yellow Alert System"

Determined to make a difference, I developed a preventive system for dysphagia, a straightforward yet life-saving approach that could reduce the risk of aspiration pneumonia in vulnerable patients.

I called it the "Yellow Alert System" or YAS—a nod to the bright yellow caution tape used at crime scenes.

Dramatic? Maybe.

But effective? Undoubtedly.

The system included an instructional bedside sign with a positional diagram I carefully designed—simple, direct, and, most importantly, practical. With the help of my dear friend Pam, I co-wrote a 200-page dysphagia manual and another instructional guide called *Eating Well*, which was distributed to patients.

The results spoke for themselves.

My system gained traction, earning me invitations to present at conferences, including the California Speech-Language-Hearing Association (CSHA). As far as I know, hospitals like Stanford Medical Center still use it today.

I also had the privilege of training medical interns at the University of California Medical Center, the VA, senior living facilities, and other care centers.

I found myself in my element—educating, advocating, and making an impact. My background in theater even turned me into an engaging (and sometimes overly animated) presenter, but hey, if it kept people's attention and helped them absorb life-saving information, I wasn't going to tone it down.

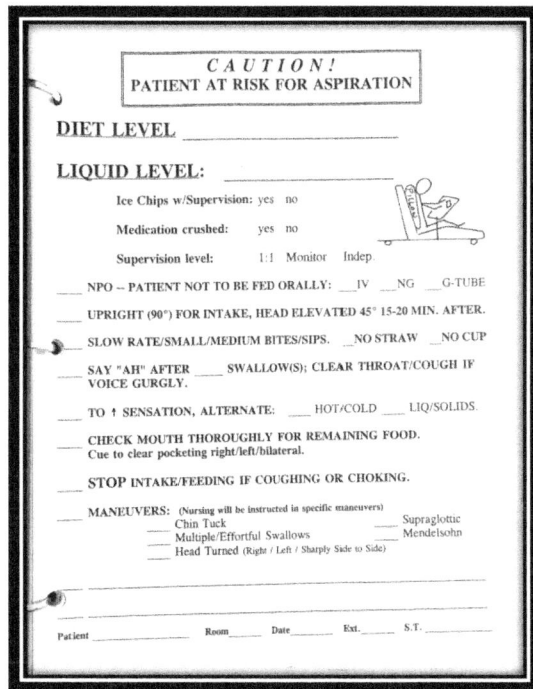

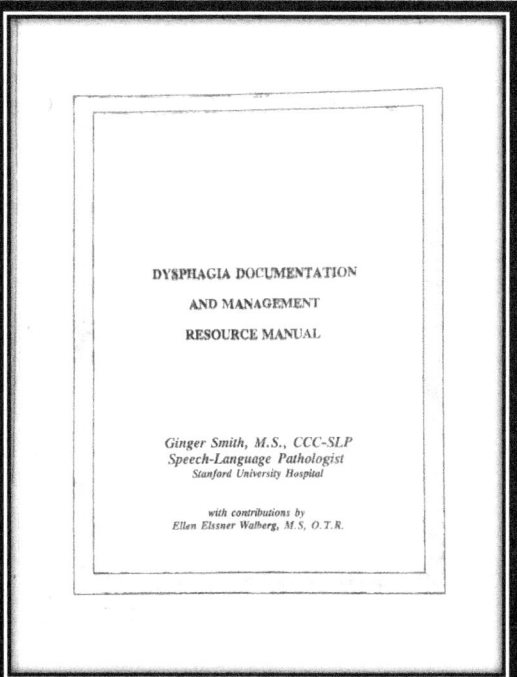

Bedside instructions for the YAS   *Cover page for the 200-page YAS Manual*

The Hidden Heroes of Healthcare

When most people hear "speech-language pathologist," they think of someone helping kids turn "wabbit" into "rabbit."

But SLPs are so much more.

We are often called the **medical detectives of the therapy world**—and for good reason. Unlike occupational or physical therapists, who must follow physician's orders, SLPs are equipped with the advanced education and clinical training to evaluate, design, implement, and write our own care plans.

This autonomy allows us to craft highly individualized treatments, helping patients regain their ability to speak, swallow, and communicate—basic human functions that most people take for granted until they're lost.

The Rising Demand for SLPs

It's no surprise that the demand for speech-language pathologists is skyrocketing, particularly in dementia and neuroscience care. With an aging population and the increasing prevalence of conditions like dementia and stroke, the need for specialists trained in cognitive communication disorders has never been greater.

According to the U.S. Bureau of Labor Statistics, the field is projected to grow by 21% through 2031—a staggering rate that highlights just how critical SLPs have become across the healthcare landscape (*What's Driving the Demand for SLP's?* | *AMN Healthcare*, 2022).

In adult healthcare settings, SLPs dedicate around 14% of their time to patients struggling with cognitive communication disorders. And their expertise extends beyond therapy sessions to caregiver counseling and support, making them an essential part of the care continuum (Lanzi et al., 2021).

But here's the problem: there aren't enough of us to meet the demand.

Despite the desperate need, the profession faces a shortage—largely due to the extensive educational and clinical requirements (*Is There a Shortage of Speech-language Pathologists?*, n.d.). Becoming an SLP isn't just a matter of getting a degree and calling it a day; it requires years of rigorous study, clinical practicums, and post-graduate fellowships before one can even begin practicing independently.

And while the research continues to highlight the profound impact SLPs have on dementia care, the challenge remains—how do we train enough specialists to keep up?

Life and Death Decisions

As an SLP, I often found myself holding life-and-death decisions in my hands.

Doctors frequently relied on me to determine whether a patient needed a nasogastric tube for feeding or if they could manage oral intake safely. In ICU settings, I was the one assessing whether someone had the ability to swallow without aspirating, a decision that could mean the difference between recovery and a fatal case of pneumonia.

It was exhilarating.

It was terrifying.

And it reinforced just how vital our work is.

But my role wasn't limited to swallowing and survival. Over time, I became an expert in treating **phono traumatic injuries** (vocal strain caused by overuse or misuse), **sarcopenia** (the gradual loss of muscle tissue), and stuttering.

And, surprisingly, my background in theater made these therapies not just effective but downright enjoyable. Who would have thought all my years on stage would serve me well in helping patients find their voices—literally and figuratively?

My Golden Era

The next two decades—starting in the 1990s—became the golden era of my professional life.

I thrived.

I climbed the ladder.

I built a career that mattered.

One of my proudest moments was being invited to Washington, DC, as a featured speaker at the first-ever conference bringing together therapists and AIDS patients. Standing at that podium, looking out at the audience, I felt an overwhelming sense of pride—not just for myself, but for the journey that had brought me there.

It was a moment that solidified everything.

I had taken the struggles, the setbacks, and the raw, messy chaos of my past and turned it into something meaningful.

Looking back, I don't see a collection of missteps. I see proof of my resilience.

From graduate school to professional triumphs, I tackled every challenge—academic, personal, medical—and transformed them into opportunities to grow.

Sometimes with honesty.

Sometimes with whiteout.

But always with determination.

CHAPTER 15: SWALLOWING SUCCESS

Speech-language pathologists are often overlooked in the medical field, but our work extends far beyond teaching kids to pronounce their "R's" correctly. We tackle **neurological disorders, strokes, traumatic brain injuries**, and even the challenges of **tracheostomies** (an opening surgically created through the neck into the trachea (windpipe) to allow air to fill the lungs) and **ventilators**—helping those who have lost their ability to communicate find a voice again.

During my time at Sequoia Hospital in Redwood City, I worked extensively in ICUs, where patients often faced complex respiratory conditions that rendered them speechless. So, I created custom communication boards, ensuring that even those tethered to life-support machines could express themselves.

One of the most critical tools in my arsenal was **video fluoroscopy**, a specialized X-ray that allowed me to assess swallowing function. Alongside radiologists, I evaluated patients, designed therapeutic exercises, and modified diets to prevent life-threatening **aspiration pneumonia**. It wasn't glamorous, but knowing that I was restoring a basic human function—the ability to eat safely—was profoundly rewarding.

The Richest Man in the World

Sequoia Hospital was known for its cardiac care, and one day, I was called in to assess a patient with mild swallowing issues. Simple enough, right?

Then I heard the kicker: "By the way, he's the richest man in the world."

I stepped into his room and instantly felt like I had wandered onto the set of a Hollywood movie. The bodyguards, handmaidens, and personal physician were enough to make anyone feel like an intruder. When I reached out to feel his throat muscles—a standard part of any swallowing assessment—one of his huge (but quite swarthy) bodyguards grabbed my arm, forbidding me from touching him.

Fine by me. I managed to assess him from a distance, confirmed that he was not in danger of choking, and promptly left—before the situation could get any weirder.

Compassion in Crisis

The most meaningful chapter of my career came in 1994 when I was assigned to the AIDS ward at Sequoia Hospital.

The epidemic was still raging, and many young men were dying alone—abandoned by their families and cast aside by a society that viewed them as outcasts. I developed a special system for those in hospice, ensuring their final moments were filled with dignity.

For those who could no longer swallow and had chosen to forego further treatment, I prepared pain medications in oral syringes and presented them ceremonially in glasses of shaved ice—a final toast to life before the medication was gently injected deep into the mouth and took effect. It was a small, humanizing touch in an otherwise mercilessly undignified disease.

I also created memory books and communication binders, helping patients and their families connect when words were no longer possible.

Outside of work, I volunteered with an AIDS organization, undergoing extensive training to provide support, care, and understanding in a world that had turned its back on these men.

A Mother's Worst Fear

In the midst of my work, I received a phone call from my youngest son, Shawn, that shattered me:

"Mom, I tested positive for HIV."

The air left my lungs.

For days, I oscillated between numbness and full-blown panic. My colleagues, many of whom had walked this road with their own patients, helped me process the devastating news.

Then, a second call came—one that rewrote the entire narrative. Shawn didn't have HIV. He had hepatitis C.

Relief, followed immediately by new fear. At the time, hepatitis C was a slow-moving killer, treated with brutal medications that carried a low success rate and horrific side effects.

I sent him $800 every month for his medication, watching helplessly as he suffered through the horrific side effects—the nausea, the exhaustion, the crushing depression. He fought like hell, and by some miracle, he won.

But fate wasn't finished with him yet.

The Legal Roller Coaster

Shawn had always been a fighter, but life seemed determined to throw him one impossible battle after another.

His first marriage had crumbled—his wife, unstable and volatile, suffered from the same anoxia at birth that had marked Shawn's own life with struggles. Their separation felt inevitable.

Then came Liz, the babysitter—young, beautiful, and drowning in her own demons. It was a chaotic relationship from the start, but out of that chaos came a little girl with a name too radiant for the storm surrounding her: Crystal Destiny.

For a brief moment, it seemed like Shawn might actually pull himself free. He achieved drug-free sobriety, committed to a live-in rehab, and for a fleeting time, his life had stability.

And then, the unthinkable happened.

Desperate to save Liz from her spiraling addiction, Shawn took matters into his own hands, trying to force her into rehab so she could finally clean up her act.

The courts called it "kidnapping" and "illegal restraint."

The good intentions were lost in translation, and suddenly, my son—the one who had fought so hard to change—was sentenced to 15 years in maximum security prison.

And because life loves irony, his cellmate was none other than <u>Larry Eyler</u>, the infamous Highway Killer.

Ty and I testified at his trial and begged for leniency, but it was no use.

I'll never forget the anguish on Shawn's face as the cuffs snapped shut around his wrists as he was led away from us into the system that would nearly swallow him whole.

For the next few years, I visited him every month, making the trip with his young son, Josh, whom I had taken in as my own.

On our first visit, I made the rookie mistake of wearing denim jeans—not realizing that in prison, <u>denim is forbidden for visitors</u>. It could be mistaken for inmate clothing.

With no time to spare, I ran to my car and grabbed the only alternative: Josh's too-tight, stinky black hockey pants.

Let's just say I made an impression.

But Shawn's story didn't end there.

With the help of a jailhouse lawyer, he fought his unjust sentence and, miraculously, was released 12 years early.

For years, he remained clean, rebuilding his life, proving that even the darkest chapters can hold redemption.

I cherish the memory of his recent surprise visit, a reminder that beneath his struggles is a man doing his best to be a loving son, father, and friend. He's made mistakes, he's faced his demons, but at his core, he is a man who loves fiercely and never stops trying.

Much of his journey—his struggles and triumphs—can be traced back to his birth anoxia, his trauma, and our family's long battle with addiction.

He's been unfairly blamed for things—my financial struggles, misunderstandings about my neurocognitive disorder—but he has forgiven me for my missteps, and for that, I am deeply, endlessly grateful.

He remains close to Crystal, despite the complicated history, and though I sometimes wrestle with guilt over how his life unfolded, one truth remains:

I am proud of the man he has become—a flawed but deeply caring person who continues to try, even when life doesn't make it easy.

The Charming Stalker

Not long after Shawn's legal battle ended, somewhere in my early 60s, and just when my life seemed to *finally* be leveling out, I found a new obsession—one I never saw coming.

 It all started with a video of Olympic ice-skating champion Brian Boitano performing while dressed head to toe in black.

Something about him—his movements, his presence, his sheer elegance on the ice—triggered a long-buried memory of my father.

The last vivid image I had of my father, apart from a fleeting glimpse from a distance in childhood, was of him standing in all black next to a pool.

And just like that, I was hooked.

I dove headfirst into the world of figure skating—taking lessons, attending every performance I could, and, well... let's just say I might have accidentally crossed the boundary from "overzealous fan" into "stalker" territory.

At one point, I tracked down where he lived.

Then, in a move straight out of a bad rom-com, I hid in the rink bathroom until it was closed for his private ice time, then emerged like an old friend who just happened to be in the area.

To his credit, Brian was gracious and polite and didn't call security.

From there, my Boitano Era only escalated.

I attended *The Phantom of the Opera* eight times—yes, eight—because Brian was backstage, waiting for Franc

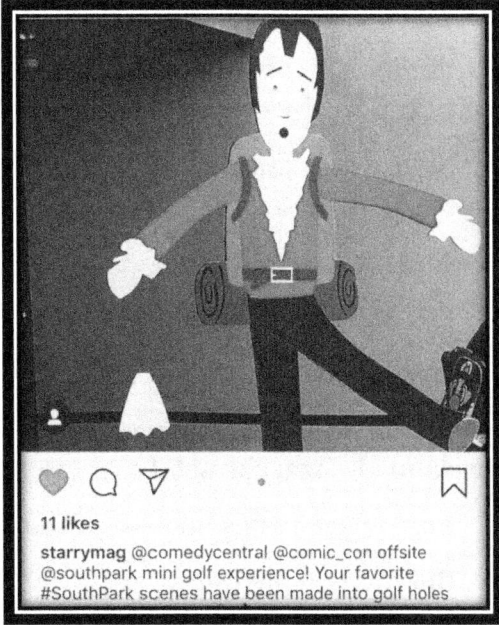

11 likes

starrymag @comedycentral @comic_con offsite @southpark mini golf experience! Your favorite #SouthPark scenes have been made into golf holes

D'Ambrosio, his partner (and the opera-singing son in *The Godfather Part III*).

Then, because casual fan gifts wouldn't cut it, I hand-crafted a cartoon magnet of his *South Park* character, complete with the *What Would Brian Boitano Do?* tagline.

Brian put it on his fridge.

That, my friends, was *my crowning achievement*.

I even met his family and gifted his mother with a tote bag I made for her, complete with silk-screened images of Brian's performances.

I also sat with his mom during his first Olympic announcing gig. We were thrilled to see Brian, who was not naturally outgoing in nature, excel in his commentary. It was like watching your introverted friend crush karaoke night.

Brian even gave me a big hug after Franc's final performance, a moment I'll treasure forever.

Skating into the Sunset (And Straight into a Wall)

Naturally, I couldn't stop there.

I joined an amateur precision skating team, despite having zero precision.

We took second place in a Las Vegas competition, which sounds impressive until you realize only two teams were competing.

Still, we performed at bat mitzvahs, birthday parties, and anywhere that needed a little sequined chaos.

Then came Halloween at the rink.

I went as a wild witch—so convincing that I scared Brian.

Josh dressed as a dead hockey player.

Ty, in a Spider-Man costume so tight, took one look in the mirror and exclaimed, "You can see I was circumcised!"

Borrowing Josh's hockey cup saved the day—and Ty's dignity.

But the real pièce de résistance?

I forgot I was on call at Kaiser and waltzed into the hospital in full witch regalia.

The doctor, ever the good sport, barely blinked as he said, "Glad you could make it, my liege."

The Fall that Ended it All

But like all good things, my skating adventures came to an end.

Neurological issues started creeping in—losing my balance, falling backward, snapping at people over trivial things.

One day, after yet another fall, I knew.

It was over.

In true dramatic fashion, I stalked off the ice for good—and by "stalked," I mean I shuffled away like a dejected penguin.

It wasn't just the end of skating. It was the end of that part of my life—the movement, the camaraderie, the ridiculousness that had made it all so much fun.

And without it, I felt adrift.

CHAPTER 16: THE POWER OF HUMANITY

As I hung up my skates, real life came crashing in.

Near the start of my SLP career, my son Shawn—struggling with his own demons—had become unable to fulfill his responsibilities as a father.

And so, his eight-year-old son, Josh, came to live with my mother and me.

In our tiny one-bedroom condo.

"Cozy" was an understatement.

Money was trickling in slower than molasses on a cold morning.

Yet Josh adapted like a champ.

He had—and still has—a personality so bright it could cut through the darkest days.

His laughter, his resilience, his ability to roll with the punches—all of it made even the toughest moments bearable.

Even when life was falling apart, even when I felt like I was coming undone, there was Josh.

He adapted like a champ, never once complaining about the tight space, the financial struggles, or the fact that he was now being raised by his grandmother—an overworked speech therapist.

Losing the One Who Held Everything Together

If I was the one keeping the lights on, my mother was the one keeping our home together.

Josh adored her—not just because she could cook the kind of meals that made you forget your troubles, but because she was his biggest cheerleader, his tutor, and his safe place.

She helped him with his homework, gave him the kind of wisdom that only grandmothers can offer, and, most of all, made him feel secure in a world that had been turned upside down.

When she passed away during his adolescence, it hit him hard.

The loss of her presence, her kindness—and, let's be honest, her cooking— left a hole that was impossible to fill.

Pairs Skating: My Ultimate (Failed) Sales Pitch

Through it all, Josh found his own escape—hockey.

But me? I had bigger dreams for him.

Not just hockey dreams.

No.

I wanted him to be a pairs skater.

And if you're wondering if this was purely because it meant more time for me in Brian Boitano's world, you are absolutely right.

So, I pitched it to him hard.

"Josh, there's a 100-to-1 ratio of girls to boys in figure skating. The girls' families pay for everything, and you'd get to hold them during lifts—with your hands in some pretty, ahem, private areas. Just think of the opportunities!"

It was my best sales pitch.

He didn't bite.

But I wasn't entirely defeated.

I insisted on teaching him some figure skating techniques, knowing that the balance, agility, and footwork would make him a better hockey player.

And, despite the occasional embarrassment of his hockey friends watching, Josh never once complained, which is truly remarkable for a teenager, if you really think about it.

Years later, those same hockey buddies admitted that my unsolicited skating lessons had actually helped him.

They had made him faster, more balanced, and more precise on the ice.

And that was a win for both of us.

Not Just an Ordinary Patient

While I was navigating the chaos at home, my career was about to take a turn I never expected.

One of the most profound moments of my time as an SLP came in 1997 when I was assigned a patient unlike any other—the renowned writer, psychologist, and spiritual teacher Ram Dass.

A devastating stroke had left him barely able to speak, and I was brought in to help.

At first, I was skeptical.

Years of phoniness from self-proclaimed "spiritual gurus" had made me cynical.

But stepping into his hospital room and meeting Richard Alpert (his birth name), the man behind _Be Here Now_, was a revelation.

This was not a fraud.

This was not an act.

This was a man who radiated pure love for humanity, even as he battled his own immense frustration.

And at that moment, I knew—this was no ordinary patient.

A Bond Beyond Therapy

We built a connection that extended far beyond our therapy sessions.

My role became more than just speech rehabilitation—I also helped his devoted followers navigate the mess that was Kaiser's hospital bureaucracy.

To keep everyone organized, I created a memory binder:

- A place to track his visitors.
- A place to document his progress.
- A place filled with affirmations of his recovery.

And, because I truly believed in his ability to heal, I told his followers something else:

"One day, he's going to write a book about this experience."

And wouldn't you know it? He **did**.

(_Still Here: Embracing Aging, Changing, and Dying_.)

A Dinner to Remember

As a thank you, Ram Dass invited me to his home in Mill Valley for dinner.

It wasn't just a meal.

It was an experience.

We sat on the floor, enjoying a simple vegetarian meal while sitar music played softly in the background.

The air was thick with peace, with gratitude, with something I can only describe as spiritual clarity.

It was a moment I never expected—and one I will never forget.

From the Typing Pool to Changing Lives

As I sat there in Ram Dass's home, I couldn't help but think about how far I had come.

Just a few years earlier, I had been clacking away in the typing pool, stuck in a job that felt so far removed from my purpose.

And now?

I was here.

A respected professional.

A speech therapist making real change.

A woman who had built something out of nothing.

My career had become my masterpiece—and every patient, every challenge, every unexpected twist was a brushstroke on the canvas of my life.

And yet, even as my career flourished, life was waiting in the wings with more challenges ahead.

Because if there's one thing I knew by now, it was this:

The universe never lets you get *too* comfortable.

CHAPTER 17: A GOOD LIFE, WITH PLENTY OF CHAPTERS

For a brief, golden stretch of time, life felt almost storybook-like.

Ty, Josh, and I were a tight-knit trio, navigating life together with a sense of adventure and camaraderie.

There were trips to Disneyland, school events to attend, and even the occasional family ice skating lesson.

Ty, ever the ambitious one, got engaged to Tanya, a brilliant and complex woman with a memory like a steel trap and an honesty that could make a saint blush.

Together, they found their passion in the therapy dog community, training their award-winning Yorkie and visiting hospitals to bring comfort to patients.

Watching them dedicate themselves to something so meaningful filled me with overwhelming pride. It was a reminder that healing often comes from the most unexpected places—sometimes in the form of a small, scrappy dog with a talent for sensing pain.

But work, for me, was just as fulfilling.

I had finally found my rhythm as an SLP, thriving in independent roles where I could work without someone constantly looking over my shoulder (because, let's be honest, I've never handled criticism well).

At Stanford University Medical Center, I poured myself into my work, but one of my favorite projects came at DeAnza College—where I worked with stroke survivors to stage a *Wizard of Oz* play.

Naturally, I cast myself as the Wicked Witch—a role I was born to play.

It was inspiring, rewarding, and—thanks to my brilliant best friend, JoAnn, who co-led the project with me—endlessly fun.

JoAnn became a beloved figure among our students, proving that generosity and intelligence are contagious. We weren't just teaching stroke survivors how to regain their voices; we were showing them that even a damaged brain can find new pathways, new ways to communicate, and new ways to exist in the world.

Later, I made an unexpected shift—working in schools.

To my surprise, I ***loved*** it.

Mentoring graduate students, guiding high schoolers interested in SLP careers—it all felt deeply meaningful.

Even now, those connections remain.

Recently, one of my former interns, Tiffany Chang, reached out, and we reconnected over lunch.

It was a reminder of just how many lives I had touched along the way—and how the ripple effect of healing can extend far beyond what we ever expect.

The Final Years of My Career: A Downpour Before the Storm

For a while, things were good.

I had achieved success, built strong relationships with patients and colleagues, and—after years of scraping by—finally had financial security.

When a condo with a breathtaking view became available next door, I jumped at the chance.

Josh, my mother, and I moved in, and I even splurged on a beautifully decorated sunroom—a small, well-earned reward.

Ty bought my old condo, making us neighbors, and for the first time in years, life felt settled and close-knit.

But good things never seem to last forever.

As I approached age 75, my family began to notice things.

At first, it was little things—subtle forgetfulness, the occasional confused expression.

Then came the money problems.

A $4,000 check to Josh—which I only recently discovered in an old checkbook.

Handing out $1,000 gifts to relatives with no memory of doing it.

Unexplained falls, moments of vacant staring, lapses in executive function.

The official diagnosis was a frontal lobe stroke with brain atrophy.

The silver lining was that my muscle strength and speech were untouched.

The downside?

Executive function is kind of important when you're trying to live, you know, as a human being.

Pushing Through—Despite it All

Despite the growing cracks in my health, I kept going.

I continued to mentor students, develop programs, and push forward in my work.

Guiding graduate students through their clinical fellowships became one of the greatest joys of my career.

But my final years as an SLP were spent working with a new group of patients—autistic middle schoolers.

It was exhausting. It was challenging. But it was incredibly rewarding.

Some students made huge breakthroughs.

Others progressed inch by painstaking inch.

But every step—big or small—was a victory.

And through it all, I developed a deep empathy for not just my students but their families—even the "helicopter parents," who, at times, made my job a bit of a nightmare.

I understood them. Their relentless advocacy made sense to me, even when they made my job harder.

In the end, we were all fighting for the same thing—a better future for these kids.

A Lunchtime Revolution

But my proudest moment at Bowditch Middle School didn't happen in the classroom.

It happened during lunch.

Before I came along, my autistic students spent their lunch alone.

Every day.

No friends. No conversations. Just isolation.

So, I decided to change that.

I opened my lunch hour to them—no structure, no expectations—just a place to sit, talk, and be *included*.

At first, only a few showed up.

Then a few more.

At first, they ate in silence, cautious, unsure of how to interact.

And then, something incredible happened.

They started talking—not just to me, but to each other.

Real conversations happened. Friendships formed.

Parents began noticing social skills they had never seen before.

What started as a quiet lunch table became a *community*—a place where these kids felt safe enough to connect.

I watched as they unlocked parts of themselves that had been waiting to be set free—a joke shared, a question asked, a simple gesture of inclusion that meant everything.

At the time, no one had ever heard of something like this.

But it worked.

Because the brain isn't just wired for survival, it's wired for **connection**.

For my efforts, I was honored with a special teacher recognition award.

But the real reward?

Watching those kids find their place in a world that often doesn't make room for them.

The Storm Clouds Gather

My mother—who had lived with me for a decade—had always been strong, resilient, the glue that held everything together.

Even in her late 80s, she seemed invincible.

But age and illness were catching up with her.

It started with a broken leg. Then spleen surgery.

And then, the worst news of all—

A diagnosis of throat cancer.

I could see it happening in real-time—her body shrinking, her strength dissolving, her mind fading in ways that reminded me of patients I had worked with for years.

I had spent decades watching brains betray their owners, unraveling in slow, cruel ways.

And now, I was watching her brain begin to shut down, too.

Her final months were unimaginably painful.

At just 85 pounds, she refused hospitalization, determined to die on her own terms.

And so, in an act of both love and desperation, I gave her a small dose of fentanyl to ease her suffering.

Within hours, she passed peacefully, surrounded by family—including Josh, who was practicing a speech about brotherhood at the time.

I had spent my career helping people regain their voices, but this was something else entirely.

This was about letting go.

And for the first time in my life, I realized—

Sometimes, the only thing left to do is surrender.

The grief was immense, but I found solace in knowing her final moments were spent at home, just as she had wished.

Looking back, I wish I had known about death doulas—an intervention I now strongly advocate for after witnessing how much comfort and dignity they can provide in such heartbreaking moments.

Because even though my mother's life had ended, something else was beginning.

A shift.

A slow, creeping unraveling of my own.

And I didn't see it yet, but my brain had already started rewiring itself in ways I couldn't control.

This wasn't just grief.

It was the beginning of something much worse.

Down the Rabbit Hole

After my mother's death, the foundation of my life—the one I had carefully built over decades of resilience and reinvention—began to crumble.

Grief hit hard, but it wasn't just grief. It was exhaustion, it was fear, it was a growing awareness that something wasn't right with me.

And then, there was the fentanyl.

It was left over from my mother's hospice care, and I told myself I'd get rid of it. Instead, I used it—convincing the hospice nurse that there was nothing left when she asked.

Seventeen years of sobriety—gone.

At first, it was just once, just to numb the pain. But it was a crack in the dam, and soon, the floodwaters came rushing in.

When the fentanyl was gone, I turned to medical marijuana, telling myself it was harmless—a natural remedy for my declining mental state.

It wasn't.

It didn't take long before I had lost more than just clarity—I had lost my teeth.

Yes, all of them.

I spent eight humiliating months without them, trying to teach speech therapy to autistic kids while grappling with cognitive decline and a dentured mouth—a combination so absurd it would have been funny if it weren't so tragic.

But the worst was yet to come.

A Call for Help, A Catastrophe Instead

One day, after three months of nightly marijuana use, I panicked at work.

I was exhausted, overwhelmed, and in desperate need of someone to talk me off the metaphorical ledge.

So, I tried calling my former psychologist at Kaiser.

I just wanted reassurance. A few calming words, maybe some perspective.

Instead, his receptionist, a social worker, decided my call sounded like suicidal ideation.

To be clear, I never mentioned a plan, a weapon, or a timeline.

I wasn't planning anything—I was just venting.

But the social worker called the cops anyway.

The police tried calling my cell—but thanks to the nonexistent reception at my school, they couldn't get through.

So, naturally, they decided to show up at my house instead.

When I didn't answer the door—because, you know, I wasn't home—they whipped out a battering ram, ready to bust in like I was a fugitive on the run.

Just as they were about to reenact an episode of *Cops*, my daughter-in-law rushed over, frantically explaining that I was at work.

And so, in full uniformed force, they marched straight into my school.

What should have been a quiet day became a public spectacle.

In full view of my coworkers, my students, and probably a few rubbernecking bystanders, they escorted me out of the building—placing me on a 5150 hold and taking me straight to a psychiatric hospital for a three-day stay.

Three days.

Three days to sit in a stark hospital room, processed like an unstable patient, all for what had been a plea for reassurance.

Needless to say, I never returned to teaching after that.

But I ***did*** make a point to go back to my office, tie up loose ends, and finish all my reports—because, apparently, even a dramatic exit doesn't exempt you from paperwork.

By December of 2015, at the age of 78, I officially retired, citing an "illness"—though the truth was far messier than that.

Honesty: The Double-Edged Sword

You might wonder ***why*** I'm sharing all of this.

Wouldn't it be easier to smooth over the messy parts? To skip the humiliating details and spare my family the embarrassment?

Sure.

But that would undermine the entire purpose of my story.

The real story.

The one where raw, painful truths create the foundation for understanding—and for helping others who are walking the same path.

Caregivers of loved ones with dementia often feel isolated, exhausted, and guilty—like they're drowning while everyone else is swimming along just fine.

I know that feeling.

I also know what it's like to be on the other side—to feel your mind slipping, to be trapped in a body that isn't cooperating, to be dismissed, misdiagnosed, or ignored.

And here's what I've learned:

Sometimes, when doctors say, "It's all in your head," they're **right**—but not in the way they're implying.

Brains don't just fail overnight.

They fight. They rewire. They look for new pathways to make sense of the world.

And sometimes, that means losing yourself before you can find yourself again.

That's why I'm telling the ugly parts of this story—the ones that don't have a neat, inspiring bow wrapped around them.

Because this is what it really looks like when a person—and their brain—is falling apart before their own eyes.

And if my story can help someone else—someone who's lost, scared, or convinced that there's no way back—then the telling of it is worth every bit of discomfort.

Wrapping Up and Moving Forward

Looking back, the final years of my career weren't just a rollercoaster, they were a free fall.

One moment, I was at the height of my profession, shaping young minds, making a difference, and mentoring future therapists. The next, I was being escorted out of my workplace, my identity as a competent, respected professional crumbling in real-time.

I had spent decades building a life—one that was rooted in resilience, ambition, and reinvention. But now, the cracks were impossible to ignore.

My memory faltered, my decisions became reckless, and my grip on reality felt more fragile than ever. I was still **me**, but I could feel myself slipping away, piece by piece.

The work that had once defined me was now behind me.

And in its place? A looming uncertainty I wasn't ready to face.

I told myself I was just tired. That if I could rest and regroup, I'd find my footing again.

But life had other plans.

Because what came next would make everything I had already survived look like a mere dress rehearsal.

The hospitals, the skilled nursing facilities, the diagnoses—until I found myself in a place I never thought I'd be.

Hospice.

Given just weeks to live.

The unraveling wasn't coming.

It was already here.

CHAPTER 18: FROM RETIREMENT TO RUIN

After my so-called retirement from Bowditch Middle School, I wasn't ready to fade into obscurity just yet. Teaching had been my life—my purpose—and I wasn't about to let it slip away.

So, I took on part-time work evaluating residents in various group homes across the area. It seemed like the perfect fit—a way to stay professionally engaged, help young adults with developmental disabilities, and maintain financial stability alongside my Social Security income.

But life, yet again, had other plans.

A Recipe for Disaster

At first, the job was rewarding. The staff respected me, the work felt meaningful, and for a moment, I thought I had found a way to keep going.

Then came the dentures.

Decades of dental neglect—fueled by an unrelenting fear of the dentist—finally caught up with me. Years of avoidance had led to gum disease, rampant oral bacteria, and, ultimately, the complete loss of my teeth.

It wasn't just about neglect, though. My fear was rooted in something real.

See, I have what they call a **fasciculating tongue** (involuntary muscle twitches in the tongue, which are often associated with neurological conditions or cranial nerve issues), and my cranial nerves are congenitally displaced—a fancy way of saying that, when I stick out my tongue, it moves in an unusual and concerning way. This condition meant that numbing agents like Novocain had to be administered in a very specific way, making dental procedures notoriously hit-or-miss when it came to pain management.

And as if that weren't enough, I also had an extreme reaction to epinephrine—a component often mixed into anesthetics to enhance their effects.

Picture this: a young me, strapped into a dental chair, screaming in sheer panic as my heart raced out of control. The feeling was terrifying, and I learned to dread every visit. To avoid a repeat of those traumatic episodes, dentists had to taper down my numbing doses, leaving me to endure procedures with far too little anesthesia.

So, I avoided the dentist for years.

Until I couldn't anymore.

By the time I faced the inevitable, dentures were the only solution.

But as it turned out, wearing dentures was its own kind of torture.

They fit poorly, rubbed my gums raw, and left me in constant pain. And in my desperation for relief, I made the worst decision possible—I turned to marijuana edibles.

At first, they seemed to help—dulling the discomfort, quieting my stress, making life more bearable. But the problem with edibles? They take too long to kick in, so I kept eating more, assuming the first dose hadn't worked.

It wasn't long before I crossed a line.

One day, I made the colossally stupid decision to show up high to work.

That was it.

I had managed to find a very fulfilling part-time job using my SLP skills at local group homes working with mentally challenged young adults, where I was well-regarded by caregivers and staff alike. But this one mistake, this one irreversible misstep, got me fired on the spot.

Just like that, the last real tether to my profession was gone.

An Entirely New Low

Losing that job was bad enough. But then came the moment that truly shattered me.

One evening, thoroughly stoned out of my mind, I sat in my chair, staring at my beloved pets, when a panicked thought coursed through me—if they needed medical care, I wouldn't even be able to drive them to the vet.

That realization landed like a punch to the gut.

I had always been independent, always the one to take charge. And now? I couldn't even trust myself to be responsible for the animals that depended on me.

I quit cold turkey that night.

No more edibles. No more "self-medicating." No more excuses.

Aside from the neuroleptics my doctors had prescribed—medications that, in hindsight, were likely a mistake—I vowed to stay completely clean.

But stopping the edibles didn't magically fix everything.

Sliding into Dysfunction

The damage was already done.

My mind felt slow; my thoughts tangled.

Post-it notes became my lifeline, scattered across my home, covering every surface, reminding me of even the simplest tasks.

And yet, despite the growing confusion, I refused to sit still.

In mid-2016, I made one last-ditch effort to reclaim some control over my life.

I started the year-long process of getting dental implants—partly because I needed them, partly because I wanted to feel like myself again.

And while waiting for my new teeth, I threw myself into volunteering.

Teaching English as a Second Language (ESL) students.

Working as a peer counselor with Peninsula Family Services. Signing up for any opportunity that would take me.

But no matter how hard I tried to stay busy, my mental fog only thickened.

Somewhere along the way, the part of my brain responsible for sending coherent messages just... checked out.

I wanted so badly to stay useful—to prove to myself and the world that I still had something to offer.

So, I tried.

I signed up as a docent at the San Francisco Zoo, thrilled at the idea of sharing my love for animals with visitors. But the quizzes were too much, the long walks too exhausting, and the mental strain unbearable.

I quit before I even really began.

Then, at an animal rescue facility, I made a rookie mistake—I left a cage open. A mistake that still makes me cringe.

At the library, my attempts to help English learners floundered because I couldn't keep up with the lesson plans.

And as a greeter at the animal shelter, I was so disoriented that I couldn't even give simple directions.

Failure after humiliating failure stacked up, leaving me confused, frustrated, and lost.

Trying to Decipher My Downward Spiral

What was happening to me?

Why was everything I once handled with ease now impossibly out of reach?

Years earlier, I had been skating, teaching, and living a life that—while imperfect—still felt full of purpose. But now? Everything was slipping away.

And the worst part was that I couldn't see it happening.

It was like watching a movie where the main character was making every wrong decision possible—except I wasn't watching it.

I was living it.

At first, I thought it was depression. That made sense. I had lost my job, my sense of purpose, and my independence in a single catastrophic year.

But this wasn't just grief or burnout.

Something *deeper* was wrong.

And when I stumbled upon a scientific journal article about **bipolar disorder**—a diagnosis I had received back in 2008—a lightning bolt of recognition hit me.

The section on manic behavior read like a checklist of my worst moments:

- **Mood swings** that flipped like a coin.
- **Risk-taking behaviors** that made no logical sense.
- **Self-harm** that I had done in the past.
- **Crushing guilt** for things I didn't even understand.
- **Periods of exhaustion and depression** so deep I felt like I was suffocating.
- **Frenzied speech**, where I would talk so fast my words tripped over themselves.
- **Erratic sleep patterns**—weeks of insomnia, followed by days where I could barely get out of bed.
- **Suicidal thoughts** that came and went like waves—sometimes crashing, sometimes retreating.

Every. Single. Symptom.

And yet... it still didn't explain *everything*.

Even as I tried to make sense of my mental decline, my physical health was taking its own nosedive.

Chronic urinary tract infections—which I later learned can cause delirium—became a regular occurrence.

My body's stress response seemed permanently stuck in overdrive.

And then there were the falls.

They became so frequent that every phone call from me sent my family into panic mode, bracing for yet another trip to the ER.

I wasn't just losing my mind.

I was losing my body.

The Financial Chaos

As my cognitive function declined, my decision-making skills took a hit—especially when it came to money.

I spent recklessly.

I gave money to anyone who "needed it."

I sent my sister $300 a month for 20 years, believing it was part of her inheritance.

I bought things in triplicate—three cat litter boxes, the same blouse in multiple sizes, anything to compensate for my fluctuating weight and confusion.

And with each purchase, I sent little notes to myself.

"Good job, Ginger. You deserve this."

Other times, the notes were more brutally honest.

"Enough is enough."

But the spending didn't stop.

It was what one writer cleverly called "Amazonamania"—an obsessive, compulsive need to fill a void with needless online shopping.

A void that couldn't actually be filled.

A Colossal Miscalculation

Then came the biggest financial misstep of my life: a step that, I found out recently, I never even *needed* to take.

My condo is my sanctuary. A one-level end unit, attached on just one side, with a gorgeous, nature-filled view of a lagoon, nestled in a peaceful cul-de-sac in a perfect-weather pocket of California.

Close to San Francisco, it was the kind of property people dream of owning.

And I bought it in the mid-90s for $100,000.

Today, it would be worth around $600,000.

In a moment of deluded desperation, without consulting anyone, I made a fateful decision.

I signed up for a reverse mortgage.

At the time, it seemed like a lifeline—a way to ease my growing financial stress. Instead, it turned out to be a predatory trap, one that I now recognize as mortgage relief fraud (at least, in my specific case).

Had my cognitive decline already been officially recognized, I never would have been allowed to sign such an agreement. But thanks to my "show timing" abilities—the uncanny knack I had honed through years of acting—I fooled the representative into believing I fully understood the terms.

I even passed the mandatory HUD-approved counseling call, a safeguard meant to protect borrowers from making uninformed financial decisions.

I performed my way right into a trap.

Because of my cognitive decline, I didn't fully grasp what I was signing up for.

And it cost me nearly all of the equity in my home.

The ability to pass that on to my family—it was gone.

(For more comprehensive information about reverse mortgages, my editor has put together a free download that can be found at this **LINK**.)

A Smile Worth its Weight in Debt

And what did I spend a big chunk of that money on? My teeth.

After losing my job and failing at volunteering, I was desperate to reinvent myself.

I needed a plan—a way to stay active, social, and relevant.

That's when inspiration struck.

I would launch a home-based speech therapy business, offering one-on-one sessions to ESL students who needed personalized support.

And, of course, if I was going to run a business, I needed to look the part.

That meant dental implants—expensive ones.

I truly believed this plan was my golden ticket. With a few clients lined up, I convinced myself that the extra income would help offset the jaw-dropping cost of my dazzling new implants. After all, who wants to learn from a speech therapist who can't flash a full set of pearly whites?

The logic seemed airtight—well, almost.

While I would love to say it was purely a practical decision, the truth is, vanity definitely had a seat at the table. These implants weren't just about work; they were about reclaiming a little bit of self-confidence. And if they came with a price tag worthy of a luxury car, so be it.

The One-Day Myth

They were advertised as a "one-day" procedure—a tagline that, in hindsight, should have come with a laugh track.

In reality, that "one day" stretched into a year-long ordeal, filled with exhaustion, setbacks, and a hospital stay thanks to a nasty bout of delirium caused by an infected tooth.

Hospital-acquired delirium, though temporary, is often overlooked—a strange, unsettling condition that can last for days or even weeks. My case cleared up after an IV antibiotic treatment, unlike the dementia-like symptoms that had lingered throughout much of my adult life.

Some speculated that my cognitive decline had been nothing more than delirium, but I knew better.

Delirium is **sudden**. Dementia is **slow.**

Delirium hits like a storm, a rapid, jarring shift caused by medication side effects, infections, or underlying medical conditions. Dementia, on the other hand, is relentless, a creeping fog that dulls everything in its path.

My symptoms had been gradual, long before the hospital stay. They didn't flare up and disappear—they built up, layer by layer until they stole my independence altogether.

But what I didn't know yet...

Was that even in that fog, my brain was still looking for a way back.

The Price of a Perfect Smile

Today, the implants look fantastic. I can eat, speak, and smile like a normal person again.

But the cost was catastrophic.

And, in some twisted way, I had to laugh at the irony—I had gone to such extraordinary lengths to rebuild my *smile* while my entire life was unraveling around me.

Yet, in some ways, it worked out.

Living in the affluent Bay Area, my condo would be running me over $3,000 a month in rent. But the reverse mortgage eliminated that burden—at least, in the short term.

Still, the dream of leaving behind a large inheritance for my family is ***gone***.

And with it, some family members disappeared too—ghosting me as efficiently as my financial stability.

Ironically, my neurocognitive disorder had already made it impossible to continue my speech practice, forcing me to give it up anyway. So, the very rationale for taking out the reverse mortgage was completely unnecessary.

And then, things got even ***worse***.

See, the reverse mortgage company had assured me I could access hundreds of thousands of dollars through a line of credit against my condo.

Desperate. Trusting. Of course, I took full advantage of the offer.

And like a slow-motion train wreck, my spending spiraled out of control and went right off the proverbial cliff.

One purchase after another, fueled by confusion, a fading grip on reality, and a desperate attempt to maintain normalcy.

Until the day the line of credit hit zero.

And all I had to show for it?

A better smile and a condo full of...*stuff*.

Years later, the last of my life savings would vanish into the black hole of care facility bills, leaving me with nothing but my monthly Social Security checks—and let's just say those don't exactly scream financial independence.

When Irony Kicks You in the You-Know-What

Here's the real kicker—the most devastating, humbling lesson of this entire ordeal.

When I signed on the dotted line for that reverse mortgage, convinced I needed the money for my new teeth, ***I already had nearly $600,000*** at my disposal.

Yes, you read that right.

Between my savings and stocks—funds I could have cashed in at any time—I already had what I needed.

But by the time Ty reminded me of this painful fact, it was too late.

The financial wrecking ball, set in motion by my neurocognitive deficits, had already done its damage.

It was a cruel joke—one that my own brain had skillfully played on me.

Collateral Damage

Looking back, I can see how my financial ruin created deep rifts within my family.

To them, it must have seemed like I had thrown everything away.

They had assumed I would leave behind something for them—a safety net, a legacy.

Instead, all they saw was a lifetime of hard work drained to nothing.

And honestly? I get it.

From the outside looking in, it must have seemed reckless. Irresponsible. Unforgivable.

But how could they possibly understand the chaos I was living through?

I was grappling with a medical condition that mimicked dementia, twisting my sense of logic and judgment beyond recognition.

I made mistakes—some big, expensive ones—but I made them in a fog of confusion and desperation.

Not exactly the kind of story you'd find in a Hallmark card.

Unraveling the Threads

By early 2018, the cracks in my mind had widened into chasms.

Then, the delusions started.

I became convinced I had **Morgellons disease**—a controversial and very rare, poorly understood skin condition.

To me, it was undeniable.

Worm-like threads seemed to be growing out of the sores on my face.

And no matter how frantically I tried to convince everyone around me...

No one believed me.

I was so certain of their presence that I documented them with the help of my grandson, having him take photos as proof.

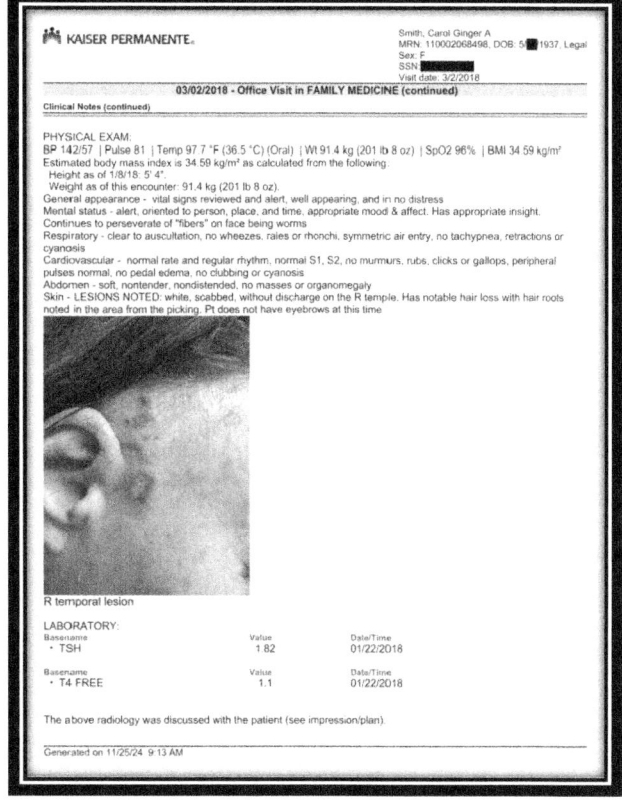

I needed validation—someone, anyone—to confirm what I was seeing.

But no one else could.

Recently, Tanya revealed the truth I had refused to see:

Those "worms" weren't worms at all.

They were simply facial hairs, more pronounced with age, that I had been obsessively pulling out—so obsessively that I had even started collecting them in what I called my "worm box."

Yes, you read that correctly.

And, yes, I carried that box everywhere.

I even showed it to people—sometimes complete strangers—offering them a glimpse at my so-called discovery like I was presenting an artifact of great importance.

Looking back, I can only imagine the horror on their faces.

The situation hit its breaking point when, in a fit of full-blown hysteria, I stormed into the Emergency Department, screaming about the worms in my skin.

My family and friends were mortified.

I was beyond reason—desperate, frantic, trapped in my own mind.

In my world, ***the worms were real***, and I needed someone to take me seriously.

But it Wasn't Malignant

At the hospital, I was diagnosed with **somatic delusional disorder**—a rare psychiatric condition in which a person firmly believes something is wrong with their body despite medical evidence to the contrary.

It wasn't just the worms.

During this period, I also suffered from **trichotillomania** (a compulsive hair-pulling disorder) and **malignant excoriation** (a disfiguring condition caused by relentless skin picking).

But when I saw the term malignant excoriation on my chart, I refused to accept it.

That phrase felt too damning, too permanent—like a label that would define me forever.

I fought back the only way I knew how: I wrote a letter.

A long, detailed, passionately argued letter to both my primary physician and dermatologist, outlining my objections and reasoning.

And shockingly, it worked.

My dermatologist revised the diagnosis to **dysesthesia** (a condition involving abnormal nerve sensations caused by misfiring signals in the central nervous system).

To me, this was a victory—proof that I wasn't just "crazy" but dealing with something biological, something real.

The Power of Validation

Something *shifted* after that moment.

For the first time, I felt like someone had listened—like my suffering had been acknowledged.

And just like that, my compulsions began to fade.

I stopped pulling out my hair.

I stopped picking at my skin.

The sores on my face began to heal.

At my worst, I had lost my eyebrows completely and rubbed bald patches into my temples, giving me the unfortunate look of a tonsured monk (tonsure is the act of shaving or cutting hair on the top of the head, often as part of monastic life).

Now, at almost 88 years old, my skin is smooth, save for the wrinkles I've earned over a long life.

But what changed?

Was it the power of validation—the realization that I was dealing with a biological disorder rather than a mental failure?

If I could bottle up whatever cured me, I'd be rich.

But the truth is, I may never fully understand what happened—only that it marked the beginning of a new chapter.

And in that chapter, I would learn something astonishing:

That even when the brain falls apart, even when it betrays you, even when doctors insist it's all in your head...

There's still a way **back**.

When You Don't Know What You Don't Know

The next couple of years—2017 and 2018—became a blur of neglect and decline.

I stopped caring for myself.

I was overweight, sedentary, and fueled by a diet of sugar and excessive coffee—the very definition of slow-motion self-destruction.

But perhaps the most dangerous part of all?

I developed **anosognosia** (a neurological condition where a person is unable to recognize their own mental health issues).

I couldn't see what was happening to me.

I was hoarding food, battling depression, and withdrawing from the world—clear precursors to my dementia diagnosis.

And yet, I didn't know.

Because when your brain betrays you, it doesn't send a memo.

It just... happens.

The world around you *shifts*, decisions feel normal when they're anything but, and before you even realize it, you've stopped living—you're just coasting toward oblivion.

But sometimes, even in that fog, the brain fights back.

It *signals*—in small, fractured ways—that something isn't right.

And for those lucky enough to listen, for those who find their way through the chaos, there's still a chance for a rewrite.

I just wasn't there yet.

Sliding Swiftly Out of Sanity

Dementia is not one-size-fits-all.

Each type comes with its own unique blend of symptoms, cognitive decline, and cruel surprises.

Mine was a bizarre and terrifying mix.

I suffered from **Capgras syndrome** (a delusion in which a person believes that someone close to them has been replaced by an identical imposter).

I also dealt with:

- **Fluctuating executive function** (inability to perform complex tasks).
- Decreased attention span.
- **Poor visual-perceptual skills** (difficulty interpreting visual information).
- Disorganized speech.
- **Micrographia** (handwriting that became painfully small and cramped).
- **Agnosia** (the inability to recognize familiar objects, people, or sounds despite normal sensory function and memory).

Physically, my body wasn't spared either.

I experienced:

- **Orthostatic hypotension** (dangerous drops in blood pressure that often caused me to collapse).

- **Sialorrhea** (excessive drooling).

- Tremors.

- An overwhelming urge to hoard and rummage.

- **Dysesthesia** (abnormal, often painful sensory distortions).

And then—my psychomotor skills began to fail.

Standing? Walking? Some days, I couldn't do *either*.

My memory issues—subtle at first—became glaring.

I started saying inappropriate things, losing my filter, and acting impulsively—a key symptom of **frontotemporal dementia (FTD)**, though my diagnosis would later shift to "unspecified dementia" with characteristics of Lewy body dementia.

Through it all, one terrifying realization gripped me:

I was disappearing from myself.

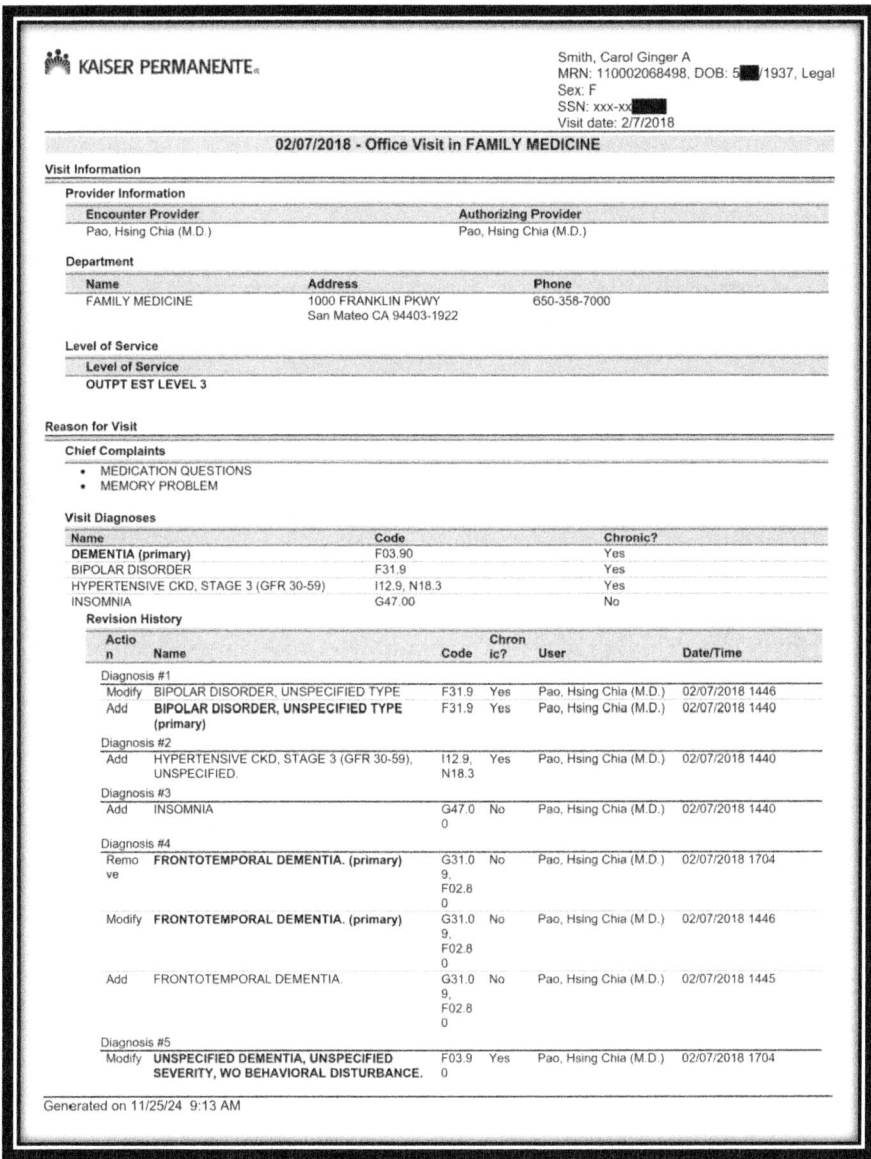

KAISER PERMANENTE Ⓡ

Smith, Carol Ginger A
MRN: 110002068498, DOB: 5██/1937, Legal
Sex: F
SSN: xxx-xx-████
Visit date: 2/7/2018

02/07/2018 - Office Visit in FAMILY MEDICINE

Visit Information

Provider Information

Encounter Provider	Authorizing Provider
Pao, Hsing Chia (M.D.)	Pao, Hsing Chia (M.D.)

Department

Name	Address	Phone
FAMILY MEDICINE	1000 FRANKLIN PKWY San Mateo CA 94403-1922	650-358-7000

Level of Service

Level of Service
OUTPT EST LEVEL 3

Reason for Visit

Chief Complaints

- MEDICATION QUESTIONS
- MEMORY PROBLEM

Visit Diagnoses

Name	Code	Chronic?
DEMENTIA (primary)	F03.90	Yes
BIPOLAR DISORDER	F31.9	Yes
HYPERTENSIVE CKD, STAGE 3 (GFR 30-59)	I12.9, N18.3	Yes
INSOMNIA	G47.00	No

Revision History

Action	Name	Code	Chronic?	User	Date/Time
Diagnosis #1					
Modify	BIPOLAR DISORDER, UNSPECIFIED TYPE	F31.9	Yes	Pao, Hsing Chia (M.D.)	02/07/2018 1446
Add	**BIPOLAR DISORDER, UNSPECIFIED TYPE (primary)**	F31.9	Yes	Pao, Hsing Chia (M.D.)	02/07/2018 1440
Diagnosis #2					
Add	HYPERTENSIVE CKD, STAGE 3 (GFR 30-59), UNSPECIFIED.	I12.9, N18.3	Yes	Pao, Hsing Chia (M.D.)	02/07/2018 1440
Diagnosis #3					
Add	INSOMNIA	G47.00	No	Pao, Hsing Chia (M.D.)	02/07/2018 1440
Diagnosis #4					
Remove	**FRONTOTEMPORAL DEMENTIA. (primary)**	G31.09, F02.80	No	Pao, Hsing Chia (M.D.)	02/07/2018 1704
Modify	**FRONTOTEMPORAL DEMENTIA. (primary)**	G31.09, F02.80	No	Pao, Hsing Chia (M.D.)	02/07/2018 1446
Add	FRONTOTEMPORAL DEMENTIA.	G31.09, F02.80	No	Pao, Hsing Chia (M.D.)	02/07/2018 1445
Diagnosis #5					
Modify	**UNSPECIFIED DEMENTIA, UNSPECIFIED SEVERITY, WO BEHAVIORAL DISTURBANCE.**	F03.90	Yes	Pao, Hsing Chia (M.D.)	02/07/2018 1704

Generated on 11/25/24 9:13 AM

Total Body Betrayal

At one point, I was also diagnosed with **medication-induced parkinsonism** (a condition caused by long-term psychiatric drug use, mimicking Parkinson's disease symptoms like tremors, stiffness, and difficulty moving).

I begged my doctor to discontinue these medications, but my pleas were ignored.

My sleep deteriorated, another hallmark of **Lewy body dementia**.

I couldn't enter REM sleep, leading to worsening hallucinations—not fleeting visions, but vivid, immersive experiences that felt real.

And then came more delusions.

Hours—sometimes days— were spent convinced that people were trying to kill me.

Reality twisted. Fiction blurred into fact.

And, as if that wasn't enough, I began losing my hearing—so severely that doctors suggested I might need a cochlear implant.

The energy required to process conversations drained what little mental capacity I had left.

And so, I retreated further.

My social interactions shrank to the occasional nod to the TV or scrolling through the endless void of the internet.

The woman who had once ridden motorcycles, who had skated across rinks with reckless joy, who had ridden through the wilderness on horseback—was now a prisoner in her own body and mind.

When It All Falls on Family

My family stepped in with every "life hack" they could think of.

Such as:

- Thinning out my hoarded collections.
- Canceling unnecessary subscriptions.
- Blocking shopping channels.
- Setting up a strict budget.
- Securing a Power of Attorney (POA) to help manage my affairs.

But dementia is *relentless*.

I lost friends—some because I pushed them away, others because they couldn't handle my decline.

I fell eight times in one year, each fall landing me in the Emergency Department, chipping away at what little independence I had left.

Finally, my family decided they were out of options.

I was placed in Grant Cuesta, a Kaiser-supported subacute facility.

By the time I arrived, I was nearly incoherent.

I couldn't follow conversations.

I couldn't trust my own thoughts.

I was barely holding on.

CHAPTER 19: SUBACUTE SURVIVAL

Before I take you deeper into my descent, let's set the record straight—*not all care facilities are created equal*. If you've never had to navigate the maze of long-term care, consider this your crash course.

Subacute Facilities: The Halfway House Between Hospital and Home

Subacute care is for people who no longer need a hospital's life-saving intervention but aren't quite ready to be set loose into the world. These facilities focus on rehab—physical, occupational, and speech therapy—for a few hours a day, with the goal of getting people back on their feet (sometimes literally).

Staff include physicians, registered nurses, and therapists, all working under the assumption that you will, eventually, leave.

Skilled Nursing Facilities (SNFs): The Long Haul

If subacute care is rehab boot camp, a skilled nursing facility is the forever home for those who need round-the-clock medical care and assistance with daily living—bathing, dressing, eating, the works. Therapy is still part of the equation, but less intense than in subacute care.

Subacute care is a stepping stone, while a skilled nursing facility is often the final destination.

Board-and-Care Homes (B&Cs): The Cozier Option

Then there are board-and-care homes, which are smaller, more home-like settings that house just a handful of residents. There are no on-site medical professionals, just caregivers helping with daily life. Think of it as assisted living without the institutional feel.

And where did I land?

Grant Cuesta. Subacute. The purgatory between hospital and home.

This is Not "Living"

My days at Grant Cuesta were a heavy haze of despair.

Roommates came and went—some of them left in body bags.

Time had no meaning. Days blurred together into an endless cycle of being propped up, wheeled around, and parked like an abandoned car near the nursing station. My "eloping behavior" (a polite way of saying I kept trying to escape despite not being able to properly operate my wheelchair) meant I was constantly under supervision—lined up alongside other drooling, vacant-eyed residents.

One man cried out for help incessantly.

Another simply stared into nothingness.

And me? I became convinced we were all being fattened up for slaughter.

Yes, I genuinely believed that patients were being selected based on their ability to eat solid food—that the ones who disappeared were either dead or had been deemed "ready." But even in the grip of this horror, I knew better than to say it out loud.

I watched. I waited. I kept my theories to myself.

And even now, looking back with a clear mind, the thought of returning to that state of decay makes me shudder.

After months of this, I started making small improvements.

I stopped babbling nonsense.

I started communicating again.

I was still in a wheelchair, but my mind was slowly returning.

During one of his visits, Ty pushed me through a park in my wheelchair. It should have been a pleasant moment of peace, a break from the fluorescent-lit misery of the facility.

Instead, I tried to convince him that the staff had a hidden second floor, where they were conducting gruesome experiments on my blood.

My hallucinations—particularly vivid ones about abused animals—felt more real than the ground beneath me.

But here's where things took a surprising turn.

Rewriting My Reality

Somewhere, buried deep under the weight of dementia, delusions, and despair, my training as a speech-language pathologist kicked in.

Years ago, I had taught patients—stroke survivors, mainly—how to reclaim control over their minds. Now, I was using the same techniques on myself.

I began to rewrite my hallucinations, turning them from horror stories into something more bearable.

A terrifying black snake became a vibrantly green, jeweled serpent. A tortured horse was rescued and sent to a sanctuary instead of dying alone.

This wasn't just me "thinking happy thoughts."

This was lucid dreaming—a practice older than written history, studied by Egyptians, Buddhists, and Native Americans, and now backed by neuroscience. And it was something I had been so dedicated to that I became really good at it.

Every night before bed, I'd perform reality checks, a technique used to train the brain to recognize when it's dreaming.

I would also meditate, setting the intention for a peaceful night's sleep, and practice progressive relaxation to ease myself into rest.

And when the hallucinations came, I changed the script.

For a brief moment, I had power again.

The Chair That Broke Me

Then came the chair incident, the most gut-wrenching moment of my entire stay.

One day, I spotted a chair in the rehab room, upholstered in a fabric that I *knew*—without a doubt—was made from the coat of my dog, Precious.

I collapsed.

I clung to the chair, sobbing and calling out, "Mama!"

But I wasn't crying for my mother.

I was crying for Precious.

For the puppies I imagined had been slaughtered before her eyes.

The pain was so real, so all-consuming, that even now, it upsets me just thinking about it.

Drugged into Submission

As my behavior grew more erratic, my doctors did what doctors often do when they don't know what else to do: *they drugged me into compliance.*

They stacked **neuroleptics** (a class of psychiatric drugs used to treat psychosis) on top of each other, ignoring the fact that these medications are specifically cautioned against for people with certain types of hallucinations.

- I became fatigued.

- I became easier to manage.

- I lost more and more control over my own mind.

My frontal lobe shut down, rerouting brain function to primitive motor control—leaving me acting impulsively, without reason, without restraint.

And worst of all? I started to believe I deserved it.

I lost friends.

I pushed people away.

I begged my grandson to euthanize me.

I had hit *below* rock bottom.

Welcome Home...Or Not

Once I had reached a point where I was considered somewhat "stable" and "manageable"—sometime around December of 2019—and in a desperate attempt to stop the clock ticking on my reverse mortgage, I returned home for a trial run at independent living.

It was an absolute *disaster*.

The chaos began almost immediately—another fall, and I was swiftly back in the ER.

My son, Ty, and two of my grandsons, Josh and Jeremy, had just picked me up for the ride home. Ty was behind the wheel, probably thinking the most challenging part of the trip would be navigating the traffic.

He had no idea what was coming.

Because somewhere between the hospital and home, I started barking like a dog.

To me, it made perfect sense.

To them? Utterly inexplicable.

From the backseat, Josh shot a wide-eyed look at Jeremy and then, like any good millennial, he discreetly pulled out his phone to record the madness. (In case you missed it earlier, there's video evidence of this moment at this **LINK**. Captions included. You're welcome.)

Once I'd finished my impromptu canine performance, I decided an explanation was in order.

See, the ER doctor had removed a piece of plastic from my mouth—a device that had been sewn in to stop me from barking. (Obviously.)

Oh, and there was also the small piece of rope stuck in my ear that was removed, which was clearly why I couldn't stop barking.

Completely logical.

The Madness Doesn't End There

But this was not a one-time event.

It happened *again* in front of Ty and Tanya when we got home—who, bless their patient souls, had no idea what to do with me.

Just like in the car with the boys earlier, I started barking—without any trigger whatsoever—and declared to Tanya:

"I'm Hitler's German Shepherd."

And when she tried to gently steer me back to reality, I doubled down:

"No, actually, I'm a gorgeous little poodle having an affair with Hitler's German Shepherd." (As if that somehow *clarified* anything.)

Meanwhile, my delusions escalated from there. My behavior became abrasive, combative, and downright hostile—especially toward Tanya, who, unfortunately, bore the brunt of it.

I was drifting further into the abyss—trapped in a fog so thick that I had no idea how lost I really was.

The Moment I Knew I Was Gone

Looking back, I've re-read some of my emails from that time.

And while I haven't found any that really match the amount of hostility my family describes, there are a few that are full of my desperate pleas.

One email to my grandson stands out:

"Help me. I don't know where I am. I don't know who I am."

I was slipping away.

And I had no way to stop it.

By late 2019, moments of clarity broke through the haze just enough for me to realize what was happening.

I felt sorrow for the pain I was causing. I apologized for my "heinous behavior."

But I still didn't understand—none of us did—that my actions weren't truly *mine*.

This was neurodegeneration.

And it was destroying me.

Here We Go Again

In January 2020, a few days before my re-admission to Grant Cuesta, things took a dramatic turn.

My hands started to tremble so violently I couldn't even hold a glass. My feet and legs swelled up like overstuffed bratwursts that had been left for way too long on the grill.

I couldn't fit into my shoes.

This led to the moment when Ty—blissfully unaware of my new symptoms—had to take me to the doctor barefoot.

Meanwhile, my dementia symptoms grew *worse*.

At this point, I had 30 out of the 34 clinical markers for **Lewy body dementia**.

There's no definitive diagnosis until autopsy, but the doctors weren't shy about throwing that term around.

Back at Grant Cuesta, the reality of my situation crashed down on me.

I felt like I was trapped in an alien environment. Confined. Isolated.

Suicidal.

The only reason I didn't act on it was because I was physically incapable of doing so.

But the mental torment of simply existing was unbearable.

OLBDA
LEWY BODY DEMENTIA ASSOCIATION

COMPREHENSIVE LBD SYMPTOM CHECKLIST

Add a check mark next to any new or concerning LBD symptoms. Write your comments or questions for the doctor in the comment field. Bring this form with you to your next appointment or send it to the doctor in advance.

2019

some *2024*

COGNITIVE SYMPTOMS	
✓ Forgetfulness	*a*
✓ Trouble with problem solving or analytical thinking	*11*
✓ Difficulty planning or keeping track of sequences (poor multi-tasking)	*11*
✓ Fluctuating levels of concentration and attention	
✓ Disorganized speech and conversation	
✓ Unexplained episodes of confusion	
✓ Difficulty with sense of direction or spatial relationships between objects	*1|*
PARKINSON'S-LIKE SYMPTOMS	
Rigidity or stiffness	
✓ Shuffling walk	*✓*
✓ Balance problems or repeated falls	
✓ Tremor	*✓*
✓ Slowness of movement	
✓ Weak voice	
✓ Change in handwriting	
Decrease or change in facial expression	
✓ Drooling	*nkd*
✓ Loss of or decreased ability to smell	*✓*
✓ Change in posture	*✓*
BEHAVIOR AND MOOD CHANGES	
✓ Hallucinations - Seeing or hearing things that are not really present	
✓ Other hallucinations (touch, smell)	
Depression	
✓ Apathy (loss of interest and drive)	
✓ Delusions (false beliefs)	
✓ Anxiety	

1

The actual form where they tracked my LBD symptoms

OLBDA
LEWY BODY DEMENTIA ASSOCIATION

2019   2024

SLEEP CONCERNS	
✓	Acting out dreams during sleep (sometimes violently), falling out of bed
✓	Excessive daytime sleepiness
✓	Insomnia ✓
✓	Restless leg syndrome
AUTONOMIC SYSTEM DYSFUNCTION	
✓	Dizziness, lightheadedness or fainting – or changes in blood pressure
✓	Sensitivity to heat and cold
	Sexual dysfunction
✓	Urinary incontinence
✓	Constipation *minimal*
✓	Unexplained blackouts or transient loss of consciousness
REACTIONS TO RECENT MEDICATION CHANGES	
	Significant improvement
	Minimal improvement
	No change
	Increased parkinsonism (stiffness, rigidity, etc.)
	Increased confusion
	Increased hallucinations
	Increased sleepiness
	Increased dizziness or fainting
COMMENTS/OTHER CONCERNS	

2

Losing Everything

Then came the final humiliation: complete *incontinence*.

I lost control of both my bladder and bowels.

I became completely immobile—unable to stand, walk, or even shift my own weight.

The staff had to use a hoist just to weigh me.

At first, I was still heavy—216 pounds when I was admitted.

But then I stopped eating. My brain stopped recognizing hunger signals.

And the weight fell off me like dead leaves.

- Late December 2019: 216 lbs.
- Late January 2020: 176 lbs.
- A few months later: 112 lbs.

At 5'3", after losing more than 100 pounds in just a few months, I was a ghost of myself.

But hey—at least it made me easier to manage.

Starvation as a Scorecard

Meals at the facility were another source of anxiety. They weren't just meals, though; they were graded.

If you ate enough, you stayed on a regular diet.

Three days of not eating? You got downgraded to mechanically softened food.

Still not eating? Pureed meals.

Still not eating? Feeding tube.

I knew what was coming.

I had worked with patients with Parkinson's and ALS. I saw where this was going.

And I was terrified.

Infection, Isolation, and One Last Attempt at Dignity

Then, an infection hit me like a train.

It was so severe, I became delirious.

They strapped me down so I wouldn't rip out my IV.

By the time I recovered, I could feed myself again.

But not for long.

One day, I begged the aides to let me do it. Just one small shred of dignity.

They refused. My tremors were too violent. My condition was too far gone.

And it crushed me.

Living with Pain No One Could See

Pain became my constant companion.

- **Spondylolisthesis** (a slipped vertebra).
- Arthritis.
- A deteriorating shoulder.

And my only pain relief was Tylenol and the occasional cortisone shot.

But the worst part was that my **aphasia** (difficulty expressing or understanding language) made it almost impossible to communicate my pain.

I was trapped.

In my body. In my mind. In my own *misery*.

The Caregivers Who Held Me Together

Through it all, the caregivers at Grant Cuesta—the nurses, aides, and staff—were the ones who kept me human.

I had once trained and worked as a homecare aide after my so-called "retirement," so I knew firsthand how relentless and grueling this work could be. Caregivers don't just help people—*they hold entire lives together*, often at the expense of their own health, sanity, and personal well-being.

And yet, despite everything—the diaper changes, the outbursts, the relentless unpredictability of my behavior—many of them treated me with remarkable kindness and patience.

Even when my condition pushed me into deeply humiliating territory.

The Real Cost of Dementia isn't Just Memory Loss

Here's the thing: It's not the physical disabilities or even the memory issues that destroy a caregiver's soul.

It's the ***disinhibited behaviors***. The moments when the person they love becomes someone they don't recognize. Some of the worst ones are:

- **Coprology** (an uncontrollable tendency to use obscene language).
- Sexually inappropriate or disturbing actions.
- **Outbursts** that feel personal but aren't.

I once read a comment in a dementia caregiver forum that stuck with me:

"I want my husband back, not this *imposter*."

That's the true grief of dementia—not just losing memories but losing the *essence* of who someone once was.

My caregivers endured the worst of it. They saw the side of me that even I couldn't recognize.

And yet, their compassion somehow pierced through the fog, anchoring me when I was lost in the deepest parts of my own mind.

Tied Down for My Own Good

I had become, to put it delicately, a handful.

A real nightmare at times.

There were days when my behavior was so erratic, combative, and unpredictable that they had no choice but to physically restrain me.

That's a special kind of humiliation, being tied down because you're a danger to yourself and others.

But looking back, I know it was necessary.

This condition had taken away my ability to regulate myself. The people around me weren't just trying to control me—they were trying to protect me from myself.

And yet, for my family, that knowledge didn't make things easier.

The Proverbial Fat Lady Started to Sing

Ty. Tanya. My grandsons.

They tried. They tried so *hard*.

But my **anosognosia** (my complete inability to recognize how sick I was) made things impossible.

Each time they placed me in a facility, they did it because they had no other choice.

But that doesn't mean it didn't break them.

Ty, in particular, was stretched to the limit. His health suffered. He was absolutely exhausted. The silent, suffocating stress of watching me unravel and not being able to fix it was becoming too much to bear.

For him, it was time to end this madness.

My caregivers—both professional and personal—paid a steep price to care for me.

And no amount of gratitude will *ever* feel like enough.

Going Off the (Bed)Rails

Then came my last major hallucination at Grant Cuesta.

And it was a wild one.

I became absolutely *convinced* that my beloved dog, Precious, was trapped somewhere in the facility—and that if I didn't act fast, something terrible was going to happen to her.

So, I did what any completely delusional person would do:

I tried to get out of bed and go save her.

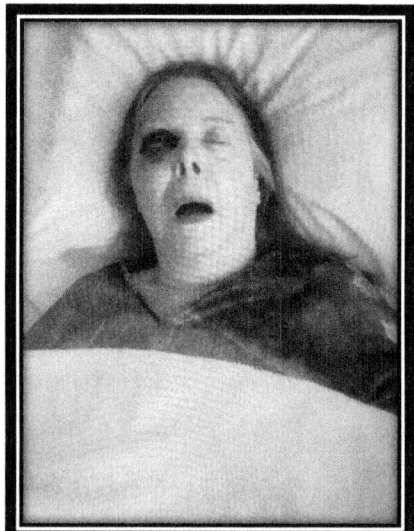

Which, given my physical condition, was a mistake.

Picture a fish flopping helplessly on dry land, trying to wriggle back into the water—that was me, attempting to stand.

Except, instead of making a grand escape, I managed to slam my right temple into the bed rail. Hard.

Cue the ER visit, the CT scan, and a giant black eye as a souvenir.

Apparently, that was the moment when the doctors officially decided Grant Cuesta wasn't the place for me anymore.

I had slipped too far down the path of deterioration.

So, they shipped me off to a board-and-care home.

But that's when things went *completely* off the rails.

The Fire Alarm Fiasco

My stay at that board-and-care facility lasted one day and one night.

That's it. (For those wondering, my editor advises against naming it to avoid legal issues.)

From the moment I arrived, I knew something was very, very wrong.

Almost all of the residents were bedbound—their feeding and urine tubes sprawled across the floor like snakes.

Except for one resident, a tiny, ancient woman who had seized control of the facility's only TV remote to watch nothing but Filipino soap operas.

When I tried to grab the remote and switch to something in English, the owner of the facility came after me with a frying pan. Yes, really!

At that point, my paranoia kicked into overdrive.

I became completely convinced that the owners were keeping these residents alive for profit—illegally sustaining them to milk money out of the system.

So, I did the only thing that made sense to me at the time.

Still trying to avoid that frying pan, I scooted my wheelchair over to the wall behind the TV and pulled the fire alarm.

Within minutes, the place was swarming with firefighters and police.

Meanwhile, I saw the owner desperately trying to unscrew the fire alarm to silence it (at least she no longer had a free hand to wield that frying pan).

I sat and watched the scene unfold, feeling proud of myself, convinced I had just led a heroic rescue mission.

But as they wheeled me out and stuck me in the back of an ambulance, I had a sinking realization.

I wasn't going to freedom. I was going back to the Emergency Department.

Again.

Ty's Breaking Point

Once the ER doctor cleared me to leave, Ty told them there was ***no way in hell*** he would send me back to that place.

When that nasty B&C owner claimed that I had tried to hit another resident, Ty dismissed her accusation immediately.

In fact, he later admitted he had a bad feeling about the owner from the start.

The first red flag? When she handed my medication box back to him instead of taking responsibility for it.

Later, more signs suggested that she, too, might have been struggling with dementia.

But by the time he realized it, it was too late.

And bringing me home was simply ***not*** an option.

Ty was completely burned out. The relentless stress of my care had already cost him 35 pounds.

He was at his limit. We both were.

Nowhere Left to Go

And so, I found myself hanging out in the Emergency Department, for ***three days***.

That's how long I was stuck there while Ty desperately searched for another facility that would take me.

The problem?

- My reputation for "bad behavior"
- The sky-high cost of my care
- Ty's refusal to let them sedate me into oblivion

Looking back, I still can't decide if I was a brave, dramatic heroine... or just a walking, talking cautionary tale wrapped in compression socks. Probably both.

And just when I thought things couldn't possibly get any worse—when I was sure the script couldn't twist any tighter—Ty found Gwen's Place.

A facility that offered a glimmer of hope.

But also, a whole new set of challenges.

Which brings us to mid-February 2020—and the start of a harrowing descent while in hospice, where everything I thought I knew about dying—

was about to be rewritten...

CHAPTER 20: THE SANCTUARY THAT WASN'T

With some help from the hospital social worker, Ty had finally secured a spot for me at Gwen's Place—an older but beautiful board-and-care home licensed for both hospice and dementia care.

He painted Gwen's as a sanctuary, a place where I could finally find some peace. He even sweetened the deal with what he knew would matter most to me:

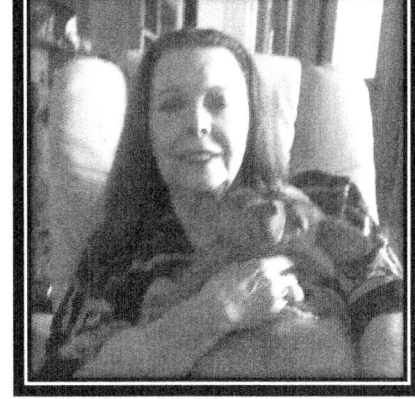

I could bring Precious.

That was all I needed to hear.

Gwen, he assured me, loved animals, had worked with therapy dogs, and would welcome my beloved companion with open arms.

For the first time in what seemed like forever, I felt something unfamiliar—

Hope.

Maybe, just maybe, this wouldn't be another house of horrors. Maybe I could have one last piece of my life with me.

But then, true to form, that tiny flicker of hope was extinguished before I even had a chance to hold on to it.

The Gut Punch

When I arrived at Gwen's, the first thing they told me was:

Precious isn't allowed.

Just like that, my last thread of sanity *snapped*.

The weight of that one moment broke me.

I felt like my heart had been ripped out of my chest—like someone had taken a piece of my soul and tossed it aside without a second thought.

I had spent so much time fighting to stay alive, holding on despite everything, believing that at least I would have *her*.

And now?

I had nothing.

Losing More Than My Dog

That night, I drifted into a fitful sleep, only to wake up and relive the horror all over again.

Precious wasn't here. Precious wouldn't be coming.

It wasn't that long ago that I lost my sweet Himalayan cat, Trek. And now this.

The grief was too much for my fractured mind to handle.

So, naturally, I started hallucinating tiny people scurrying around my bed, cleaning.

I blinked. Looked again. Yep, still there.

I sat up, bewildered, and announced:

"What's going on here?! We can't afford to pay all these tiny people!"

The absurdity of it was almost comical—except it wasn't.

It was a sign of just how far gone I was.

And yet, even in that bizarre moment, I knew:

Something inside me had broken for good.

Reality? A Delusion? Who Even Knows Anymore?

Looking back now, I have to wonder—

Was I ever *actually* promised that Precious could come?

Was that something Ty truly believed, or was it just another delusion of mine—a desperate attempt to make this new place seem less unbearable?

I don't know. I may never know.

But the pain of losing that hope?

That was real. And it still is.

Instead of Precious, the only dog in sight was Gwen's ancient Chihuahua, who took one look at me, my wheelchair, my broken body, my broken mind, and decided—

Nope.

He kept his distance, avoiding me like I was a ticking time bomb.

Honestly? It was probably a fair assessment.

But that tiny dog's wide-eyed fear of me only made me feel even more isolated, discarded, and unwanted.

They say dementia is the "long goodbye"—but losing Precious felt like a sudden, violent severance.

A sharp, unrelenting pain that hasn't left me since.

Granny Drop

February 18th, 2020.

That's when I officially arrived at Gwen's Place.

And from the moment I was wheeled inside, I felt it—that suffocating, heavy fog of hopelessness.

I was drowning in despair, barely holding on.

To make matters worse, the world outside was starting to shut down. The pandemic loomed over everything, tightening the walls around me and amplifying my isolation.

And then, there was the dramatic weight loss.

Over the past month, my body had wasted away.

Ty and Tanya—still trying to keep me alive—visited occasionally, bringing my favorite foods to tempt me into eating.

One day, they even showed up with my favorite McDonald's meal, the holy grail of comfort food.

I took one look at it and turned away.

They tried again and again. Different meals, different bribes, begging me to eat.

Nothing worked.

Then, in March, the visits stopped altogether.

COVID restrictions locked the doors, cutting me off from everyone I knew.

I understand it now.

But back then?

I felt abandoned.

Who Am I? Where Am I? Do I Even Exist?

With no visitors and no connection to the outside world, paranoia took root in my mind like a fast-growing weed, strangling what was left of my grip on reality.

I became certain—beyond a shadow of a doubt—that I had fallen victim to a legendary "granny drop."

If you don't know the term, it refers to the heartbreaking act of abandoning an elderly relative in a care facility and never coming back.

And that's exactly what I thought Ty had done.

Left me here.

Made sure I had no identification.

No way to be traced back to my family.

No wallet. No address book. No cell phone. No ID.

Nothing.

I wasn't even sure what my own name was anymore, let alone my home address.

I had no past, no proof that I had ever existed outside of this place.

And in my crumbling mind, it wasn't just neglect—it was deliberate.

Paranoia Took Over

The fear didn't stop there.

I became convinced that everyone around me—family, friends, even my caregivers—was plotting against me.

That they were trying to hurt me.

That this wasn't just a nursing home—it was a trap.

It didn't matter that the rational part of me had long since disappeared—the fear was *real*.

And when fear takes over?

You trust no one.

Because this chapter of my life—this slow descent into isolation and oblivion—was far from over.

A Room Full of Emptiness

Gwen's Place was a paradox—a home caught between life and void.

The main areas were cluttered with statues, overgrown plants, and Renaissance paintings depicting macabre, haunting scenes. It was as if the house itself couldn't decide whether it was a cozy refuge or a gothic mausoleum.

And then, there was my room.

Compared to the overwhelming chaos of the house, my space was a whitewashed void—a soulless, sterile box. No warmth. No color. No trace of life.

The only decorations were two grim paintings of a boy peering at me from behind a tree. His eyes seemed to follow me wherever I moved, their presence as unsettling as my own fractured mind.

The longer I stared at them, the more I became certain—

I was the boy.

And I was being hunted.

A Tree Becomes My Only Friend

Beyond my tiny window, a scraggly tree stood alone, its bare, twisted branches reaching for something it would never touch.

I spent hours staring at it.

Naming its leaves.

Inventing stories about its branches.

Assigning triumphs and tragedies to its existence because it was the only thing I had left to connect with.

The silence within Gwen's wasn't just an absence of noise—it was a tangible, living thing, pressing against me like an unseen force.

No cars. No voices. Not even the hum of distant life.

Just the faint squish of a caregiver's shoes on linoleum and the astringent, suffocating smell of cleaning products.

The air was dead—void of warmth, void of comfort.

Fully immersed in **sensory deprivation**, my brain began to devour itself.

Starved for Reality, My Mind Created its Own

I wasn't just alone—I was adrift.

With no sights, no sounds, and no connection to the world, my brain started filling in the blanks.

Hallucinations. Memory lapses. Fractured realities.

One day, I was just another patient in a room.

The next? I was the boy in the painting—hiding behind the tree, shotgun in hand, waiting for an unseen enemy to find me.

Was it real? No.

Did it feel real? *Absolutely.*

With no daily sounds to mark time, my memory unraveled, blurring the lines between what was real and what was imagined.

The Pandemic's Grip Tightens

I should probably mention something important here—

When I first arrived at Gwen's, the care was actually excellent.

The staff was kind, the facility was clean, and the residents—though very ill—were treated with dignity.

But I was too lost in my own fog to fully grasp it.

Communication was a mountain I couldn't climb.

Words failed me. Energy failed me. My own mind failed me.

And when COVID hit, it was like a storm cloud descended over the entire house.

One by One, They Disappeared

At first, it was just a shift in the atmosphere.

A little less laughter in the hallways. A few more closed doors than before.

Then, the deaths started.

One by one, the residents began to vanish, swallowed by the silent, aching void of the pandemic.

I was too dissociated to fully process what was happening.

But I felt it.

Each death left a hole in the house, like furniture being slowly removed from a room until all that's left are the echoes.

My Own Private Solitary Confinement

I was so deep inside my dissociative state that I had no idea what was going on beyond my own four walls.

The news? The rising death toll? The world in chaos?

Might as well have been a whisper on the wind—something unreal, distant, untouchable.

So, when Ty told me that he wouldn't be able to visit for at least two months due to shelter-in-place orders, I didn't believe him.

Too convenient.

It was easier to believe that I had been abandoned—that the excuse of a "pandemic" was just a polite way of saying they were done with me.

And so, I sank further.

Trapped in a Prison of Silence

I had no television to distract me. No phone to reach out to anyone.

No way to communicate, thanks to a brutal combination of:

- **Aphasia** (a condition that steals your ability to express or understand language).
- **Cognitive agnosia** (a disorder that makes recognizing and interpreting information nearly impossible).

I was trapped inside my own head, screaming with no way to be heard.

And my room—that sterile white box—felt like a prison cell.

If I begged or screamed, maybe someone would crack the door open slightly—a momentary sliver of human connection before they disappeared again.

But mostly, I was left in crushing solitude.

Alone.

The Moment it All Became Real

For months, I had been trapped in my own delusions.

But then—something shattered the illusion.

One day, I was being wheeled through the parlor room on my way to a doctor's appointment when we passed a television.

On the screen, I saw people in masks being escorted off buses.

A headline flashed across the screen:

"Passengers detained due to COVID-19."

And, at that moment, I felt relief and horror.

At the same time.

Reality Hits Like a Freight Train

Relief, because it meant my son hadn't lied to me.

The lockdown was real. The isolation was real.

The whole world was unraveling, not just my mind.

And *horror,* because this meant the nightmare wasn't just mine—it belonged to everyone.

For the first time, I understood that the world beyond my room, my hallucinations, and my paranoia was in a crisis of its own.

And that didn't make me feel better.

It made everything *so much worse.*

Back to My Cage

After that fleeting moment of clarity—and after being wheeled back to my room from my doctor's appointment—the walls seemed to close in even tighter than before.

I wasn't just a forgotten patient in an empty house anymore.

I was a prisoner in a world that was falling apart.

And the door to my room—so often shut—became my only connection to the life I was slipping away from.

I begged for them to leave it open, just so I could hear something— *anything*—to remind me I wasn't the last person on Earth.

Most days, I just sat in the silence, staring at the white walls, drowning in my own crumbling mind, waiting for *something* to break the monotony.

And then?

The hallucinations got even ***worse***.

Capgras syndrome entered the picture like a bull in a china shop.

The Imposters Arrive

Sometime in the summer of 2020, a new horror took hold of my mind—one that even my worst delusions hadn't prepared me for: Capgras syndrome.

For those lucky enough ***not*** to be familiar with it, **Capgras syndrome** is a delusion where you become absolutely convinced that someone close to you has been replaced by an identical imposter.

And just like that, the people around me—caregivers, nurses, even my own family in memories—became frauds, strangers wearing the faces of people I once trusted.

At first, I fixated on the medical director.

Now, to be fair, he was barely a presence at Gwen's to begin with—just someone who completed a checkbox for Medicare paperwork, swooping in occasionally to maintain the illusion of oversight.

But in my twisted, paranoia-drenched mind, he wasn't just negligent—he was an imposter.

And I wasn't about to keep quiet about it.

Sounding the Proverbial Alarm

I took it upon myself to warn everyone. Loudly. Repeatedly.

I accused him of deception at the top of my lungs, warning anyone who would listen that the doctor was a fraud—a danger to us all.

Then, spotting a young student nurse, I pulled her aside, whispering my urgent warning like I was uncovering a deep conspiracy:

"Stay far away from him. He's not who he says he is."

The poor girl looked at me with a mix of politeness and pure horror, caught between her training to be professional and the reality of dealing with a delusional woman in a wheelchair screaming about body-snatching doctors.

Eventually, another aide had to remove me from the situation—probably before I could do any more damage.

But the paranoia didn't end with the doctor.

The Body Beneath My Skin

At some point, my mind decided that one delusion wasn't enough.

I wasn't just surrounded by imposters—I *was* one, too.

There was another body living beneath mine.

Hidden, but undeniably there.

I could feel it under my skin, trapped, waiting to be discovered.

I begged Gwen and my hospice nurse to tell me what was happening to me.

When they finally told me the probable truth—that I had **Lewy body dementia**—the words hit me like a punch to the throat.

I froze.

Knowing Too Much Can Be a Curse

Here's the problem with being a speech-language pathologist who has worked with dementia patients:

I already knew too much.

I knew what Lewy body dementia (LBD) meant.

I knew it wasn't just fatal—it was devastating.

It meant:

- The disappearance of **social filters**
- Rapidly declining cognitive function
- Relentless hallucinations

It meant a slow descent into a waking nightmare.

It meant losing my grip on reality piece by piece until there was nothing left of me to save.

I begged whatever was left of my rational mind not to let this be true.

I pleaded to whatever force controlled my fate:

"Please, not this. Anything but this."

But my hallucinations didn't care about my pleas.

They had other plans.

Birds, Butterflies, and Waiting to be Rescued

Some of my hallucinations were almost whimsical.

I saw birds and butterflies, their vibrant colors dancing in front of me like some surreal, cartoonish dream.

But even those moments felt **off**—like something scripted for an audience that wasn't really there.

They weren't peaceful visions.

They felt unnervingly artificial—like watching a punch-drunk boxer stumbling around a ring, unaware that the fight was already over.

Then, there were the *darker* hallucinations.

The ones that gripped me consumed me and became my new reality.

I wasn't just imagining animals in need of rescue—I *was* the animal.

Trapped.

Helpless.

Waiting for someone to save me from an unseen tormentor.

The line between my hallucinations and my own fractured existence blurred until I wasn't sure which version of suffering was real.

Falling Apart at the Seams

Physically, I had become unrecognizable.

My body—once well-fed, once strong—was now wrapped in a size 22 muumuu, barely held together by safety pins, drowning me in its tent-like folds.

It was absurd—a body once too large for me, now barely clinging to my frame.

An unsettling symbol of how little control I had left.

There were days—far too many—when I was left for hours in soiled diapers, immobilized, unable to even feed myself.

Some days, I lay in my own urine for hours upon hours.

I'd once been a professional, a caregiver.

Now, I was a body waiting to be managed.

A patient tolerated rather than tended to.

And with no real mental stimulation, my frayed mind tried to fill the void in some of the worst ways possible.

- Compulsively picking at my skin, leaving it raw.

- Bloodying my nose from endless, mindless picking and scratching.

- Engaging in... let's call it 'groin amorousness' to the point of causing an open wound near my lady parts.

(And let's be honest—being left in a soiled diaper for half a day didn't exactly help the infection situation down there.)

At night, it got even worse.

- **Sexsomnia** (performing sexual behaviors in my sleep).

- **Scatology** (playing with feces because, apparently, my brain was now determined to strip me of *every* last shred of dignity).

My body was a stranger to me.

My own mind had turned into an enemy.

By this point in my life, visitors were nonexistent. My friends were gone.

My only real human interaction was with visiting nurses, who showed up sporadically, offering only the barest glimpse of human connection.

Most of my waking hours were spent:

- Lying motionless in bed.

- Trapped in my own head.

- Too drained to engage with the world.

Even my brief moments outside my room weren't much of a relief.

The parlor, where they sometimes wheeled me, was a windowless void—no natural light, no life, just another prison cell in a house that felt like a tomb.

Hospice: The Business of Dying

By the time I arrived at Gwen's Place back in February, the Medicare paperwork had already been signed, and I had been officially placed in hospice care.

My prognosis? Just weeks to live.

To qualify, two doctors had to certify that I had less than six months left. That meant no more curative treatments, no more hospitals, and no more medical interventions.

From this point forward, the goal wasn't survival—it was comfort.

Hospice is often painted as a compassionate, dignified farewell, a way to ease suffering in the final stretch of life. And in theory? That's true.

But, in reality, it's an industry.

An industry where over 70% of providers—including Gwen's—are for-profit businesses, with minimal oversight ensuring quality care (*FastStats,* n.d).

Dying, it turns out, can be very lucrative.

The Great Hospice Hand-Off

When someone enters hospice, the focus shifts entirely:

- No more endless tests.
- No more futile treatments.
- No more aggressive interventions to "prolong" the inevitable.

Hospitals exist to **_treat and heal_**. Hospice exists to **_ease the exit_**.

Think of it like a relay race—the hospital passes the baton to hospice, whose job is to ensure that the final chapter is one of comfort, dignity, and pain relief.

At least, that's the *idea*.

Hospice (often funded by taxpayers through Medicare) covers the essentials:

- Wheelchairs.
- Diapers.
- Nurses.
- Social workers.
- Clergy.

But here's the catch:

While hospice provides resources, much of the actual caregiving falls on family members.

During the pandemic, when professional caregivers were scarce, families were left scrambling to become dementia experts overnight—with little guidance and even less support.

Removing All Curative Meds

Before hospice, I had been juggling a revolving door of prescriptions—about twenty different medications, if you counted the over-the-counter ones.

But once I started on "comfort care," that list was cut to the bone.

Gone were:

- **Psychotropic drugs** (psychoactive substances used to treat mental illnesses by affecting the chemical makeup of the brain and nervous system).

- Benzodiazepines (anxiety meds).

- **Atypical antipsychotics** (medications used to treat mental health conditions, particularly psychosis and schizophrenia).

I had officially been classified as "actively dying"—a term hospice uses for those in the final stages of life.

My organs were shutting down, and my medical records reflected it:

- **Orthostatic hypotension** (blood pressure so low I nearly blacked out when sitting up).

- **Paradoxical agitation** (restless and anxious despite sedation).

- **Parkinsonian somnolence** (so exhausted, it felt like I was swimming in wet cement).

- **Terminal restlessness** (my body's last-ditch effort to fight the inevitable).

- A weak pulse, decreased consciousness, and terminal anorexia (when my body stopped sending hunger signals to my brain).

In hospice terms, I was in the home stretch.

Where the Hell Were My Painkillers?

Here's what no one tells you about comfort care:

Just because you're dying doesn't mean they hand you unlimited painkillers.

I had naively assumed that, once in hospice, I'd be given as much pain medication as I could ever possibly want—unlimited access to whatever I needed to escape the relentless, gnawing pain that had been my constant and oh-so-stubborn companion.

I imagined a world where pain could be erased at will, where relief was just a pill away.

Instead, pain meds were rationed, handed out sparingly, and always under strict oversight.

It wasn't the endless morphine drip of my dreams—it was a tightly controlled, bureaucratic nightmare.

And believe me, I suffered immensely because of it.

Terminal Restlessness: The Final Agony

For those unfamiliar, **terminal restlessness** is the body's final rebellion.

It's a cruel, chaotic state of:

- Agitation
- Delirium
- Moaning and pulling at bed sheets
- **An overwhelming urge to "get up,"** even when the body is too weak to move

It's as if the mind and body are caught in a brutal tug-of-war—desperate to fight, even as the body is giving out.

The causes are a toxic mix of:

- Metabolic changes
- Decreased oxygen to the brain
- Medication side effects
- Unresolved emotional or spiritual distress

But no matter *why* it happens, the result is the same:

It's devastating to witness—and even worse to experience.

For many families, it's the moment when they truly realize:

This is *the end*.

Dying Alone: The Ultimate Cruelty

As if **terminal restlessness** wasn't already unbearable, the pandemic made it even worse.

Family members weren't allowed to visit.

They couldn't hold my hand.

They couldn't sit by my side.

They couldn't offer a shred of comfort as I slipped closer to what I thought were my final days.

The thought of dying alone, without the warmth of my loved ones, was almost too much to bear.

I felt *trapped* inside a virtual locked-in state:

- Completely immobilized
- Motionless
- Unable to scoot or adjust myself in bed

Instead, my body slumped into a grotesque "Lewy lean," tilting to one side—a signature hallmark of my condition.

My Body: A Betrayal in Slow Motion

As "the end" approached, communication was nearly impossible.

I had become:

- **Aphonic** (unable to produce speech).
- **Dysphagic** (unable to swallow).

Even yes or no responses were a struggle.

Most of the time, I simply sat there, staring into space, drooling, trapped in my own mind.

Hallucinations flickered in and out, teasing me with fragments of a reality that no longer existed.

And my body was giving up, piece by crumbling piece.

Preparing for Death

I was so close to death that my family had already made their peace with it.

They had taken steps to prepare:

- Paid for my cremation
- Stripped my condo of furniture and decor
- Sorted through my belongings

It was as if my life had already been dismantled before I had even left it.

Tanya recently admitted that they had been given a "hospice kit"—a no-nonsense guide filled with checklists and to-do items for families preparing for the inevitable.

And then, they learned the harshest reality of all:

Because of the reverse mortgage, they had only two months after my passing to:

- Sell my condo
- Buy it themselves
- Or lose it entirely to the lender

No grace period. No extensions. Just *gone*.

Which is why they had started clearing out my things before I had officially kicked the bucket.

After all, I had been placed in hospice care to die…

But what does "actively dying" *actually* look like?

What does it feel like to be at the end—to exist in the void between life and death?

Let me take you there. As caregivers and loved ones, I believe it's important to understand what a typical day feels like to the one experiencing it.

Step by step.

Hour by hour.

Into the abyss of hospice, where time warps, dignity crumbles, and the body fights a battle it was never meant to win.

CHAPTER 21: A DAY IN THE ABYSS OF HOSPICE

6:00 AM: I can't sleep. I don't really sleep anymore. My body is restless, but I don't have the strength to move. I've been in hospice for months now, my fragile frame barely clinging to life after losing over a hundred pounds.

I didn't just lose weight—I lost the will to eat, the will to exist.

My body is wasting away, collapsing in on itself, but no one seems alarmed.

They call it **cachexia**.

I call it disappearing.

7:00 AM: Tony should be here by now.

He's my CNA, my only lifeline in this place. But I wait and wait.

Nothing.

I've been bedridden since I got here, unable to hold a spoon, unable to lift a glass to my lips.

Months ago, they told me I probably had Lewy body dementia, but the doctors had waffled between diagnoses for years—first Frontotemporal dementia, then "unspecified dementia," when my symptoms blurred the lines between the two.

I was in a skilled nursing facility first, then placed here, under hospice watch.

They don't expect me to leave this place alive.

7:30 AM: Still no Tony.

Something worse than hunger twists in my gut.

I feel it before I smell it.

A warm, sticky mess spreads beneath me. Diarrhea.

I am doubly incontinent, trapped in a soiled diaper, my raw skin burning from the dampness.

A new abrasion stings between my legs, another wound my body won't have the strength to fight.

I try to mumble for help, but my words tangle in my mouth. I try to scream, but my voice is barely above a whisper, swallowed by these indifferent walls.

No one comes.

Tony must be sleeping—somewhere in this too-big house—unaware.

8:00 AM: Panic sets in.

My thoughts slip away from me, scattered and fragmented.

What if no one comes? What if this is how it ends?

The undulating bed—a Medicare perk meant to keep bedsores at bay—feels like it's trying to swallow me whole.

But that's *impossible...* right?

I blink.

The walls shimmer.

Hallucinations. Again.

My body is failing, and my mind is twisting reality into something crueler than the truth.

9:00 AM: Footsteps.

A quiet squeak of rubber soles on linoleum.

Tony.

Relief floods me, but when he enters, he barely glances my way.

No greeting. No kindness.

Just a mechanical nod before getting to work.

I am *desperate* for connection, but I get *nothing*.

COVID-19 has sealed me away from the world, from my family.

No visitors. Just the staff—when they remember me.

9:15 AM: Tony cleans me up.

There's no judgment, no disgust, just clinical efficiency.

For that, I am grateful.

But, God, how I wish he would say *something*.

Just a simple *"You're okay."* Or *"I've got you."*

Anything to remind me that I am still a person, not just a task to complete.

But even when my caregivers *do* speak, their words are *lost* to me.

The COVID masks hide their mouths, making it impossible to read their lips.

I strain to understand, but all I hear is muffled sound, distant and blurred like I'm trapped behind glass.

The silence isn't just around me—it's *inside me* now.

9:45 AM: Breakfast arrives.

I refuse it.

The eggs are pureed into something unrecognizable, something alien.

I choke on solids now, my swallowing reflex as broken as the rest of me.

But that's not why I won't eat.

The food is *lava* to me—molten, dangerous, impossible to touch.

My mind has turned nourishment into a threat, and no one understands.

They think I'm just being stubborn.

10:00 AM: They close the door.

I had hoped they would leave it open, just a crack.

They don't.

I am in solitary confinement, forgotten again.

11:00 AM: Pain meds.

Too *little*. Too *late*.

I'll later find out that, before hospice, I was on *twenty* different medications—psychotropics, antipsychotics, and curative drugs ripped away overnight.

No one asked. No one explained.

They just did whatever some piece of paper told them to do.

11:30 AM: A visitor.

A real, human **_visitor_**.

The social worker.

She only comes every few weeks, but the sound of her voice almost makes me cry.

Someone is here. Someone sees me.

She looks me over and fills out a form.

Then she leaves. And I am alone again.

No cell phone. No TV. No music.

Just... **_nothing_**.

12:00 PM: Tony lifts me into my wheelchair. My feet never touch the floor.

I don't exist outside this bed, this chair, this room.

They try to get liquids in me.

My stomach revolts, and I vomit.

The aides yell—as if I'm doing this on purpose.

One of them pinches my nose, forcing the drink down.

But I am too sick.

They give up and wheel me back to my stark, white-walled prison.

12:30 PM: The pain returns. A dull throb, growing sharper.

I can't tell them where it hurts.

I can't tell them anything.

My brain _refuses_ to form the words.

They don't notice my distress until I start to writhe—my body betraying me in the only way it can.

Finally, they give me more pain meds.

But instead of relief, I sink deeper—trapped between exhaustion and restless agitation.

1:00 PM: A phone call.

Gwen smiles as she brings the receiver to my ear.

A family member? A friend?

I am thrilled—someone is checking on me!

But I can't hold the phone.

I can't respond.

They talk.

I try to listen, but without my hearing aids, all I hear are garbled noises.

Do they know how much I *need* them?

Do they know I feel **abandoned**?

The words blur together, lost in my deafened ears.

I try to form a coherent response, but my lips and tongue betray me.

Within less than a minute, the caller gives up.

The phone clicks.

And my world falls silent once again.

2:00 PM: My breathing is shallow.

I try to curl up in the fetal position, seeking some small measure of comfort, but my body won't cooperate.

I am too weak, too frail, too *broken*.

The tiny window in my room lets in just a sliver of light, a narrow reminder that a world still exists beyond these walls.

I stare at it, watching the faint glow shift across the floor.

I wonder:

Does anyone even remember that I *exist*?

3:00 PM: The nurse practitioner arrives. She is kind.

She checks my vitals, her hands gentle as she measures my scrawny arm against my emaciated frame. She seems to talk softly to herself.

I am too drowsy to hold her gaze, but I manage to smile at her.

She smiles back.

Then she leaves.

And I am alone again.

3:30 PM: Diaper change. Cleanup. Silent Tony.

4:00 PM: I wish I could read something.

I used to *devour* books.

I used to live in stories, in knowledge, in words that shaped entire worlds inside my mind.

But not anymore.

Now, my eyes glaze over the pages, my brain unable to grasp the meaning of the words.

The sentences blur and scatter, dissolving into nothing.

I just lie here, hour after hour, my mind unraveling with every moment of stillness.

And the worst part? I *know* what this means.

As a former speech-language pathologist, I know that with no stimulation, my brain is *dying faster*.

I know that I am fading away, and there is nothing I can do to stop it.

6:00 PM: One last attempt at eating.

Nope. Not happening.

My body rejects the idea of food before I even try.

More pain meds to make me "comfortable" until the morning shift-change.

Comfortable. That's the word they use in the hospice world.

But is this *comfort*?

I wonder if withdrawing my curative drugs was really the best choice.

Were the side effects of those medications truly worse than this existence?

I'll never know.

8:00 PM: Final diaper change. Lights out.

I am exhausted, but my mind *won't stop.*

I wonder if I'll hallucinate tonight—if shadowy figures will crawl from the walls to keep me company, or if I'll become a Clydesdale or jeweled green snake again.

Maybe this is it.

Maybe tonight is the night I let go.

Maybe tomorrow, no one will have to clean me up or force food down my throat—or pretend to care.

Maybe, for the first time in a long time,

I'll be free.

CHAPTER 22: AWAKENING TO SOMETHING VERY UNEXPECTED

Hospice had done everything but write my obituary.

I had been stripped of medications, left to waste away in a bed I could barely move in, in a body that no longer obeyed me. The world had already begun erasing me—my belongings were gone, my voice was unheard, and my days blurred into a slow, silent march toward nothingness.

And yet... August came.

I was still here.

At first, it felt like a cruel oversight, as if death had accidentally skipped over me and moved on to more pressing business. But then something happened— something extraordinary, something *impossible*.

One ever-silent morning, while lying in the profound stillness of oblivion, I **died**.

Well, at least I *thought* I had died. Not in a dramatic, movie-scene kind of way—but in a deep, undeniable, soul-level knowing. One moment I was in unbearable pain... and the next, it was gone.

Instead of that stereotypical "tunnel of light" people always talk about, I found myself floating in a sky so dark and deep it was almost glowing—a velvet blue expanse, speckled with endless stars that pulsed with something like... knowing.

There was no body, no weight, no confusion. Just me—or maybe, what was left of me—hovering in this eternal stillness. And for the first time in what felt like forever, I wasn't afraid. I wasn't in pain. I wasn't trying to survive.

I was simply *free*.

And then... it spoke. Not out loud, not in words I could hear, but in a clarity that thundered through me like truth itself:

"It's not your time yet. You need to go back. There are others who need your help."

Suddenly, I had a mission. A reason. A purpose that felt far bigger than me.

And before I could argue (and oh, how I wanted to argue), I was falling. Not tumbling or flailing, just... being pulled. Back. Down. Into the broken shell I had left behind.

Except now, I was changed.

Because I hadn't just brushed up against death—I had danced in the stars with it... and been told to *get back to work*.

The Shift

Something inside me **clicked**.

Like a switch being flipped, like a circuit that had long been broken suddenly sparking to life again.

For months, I had been waiting to die.

Now, I realized that maybe—just maybe—there was still something left for me to do.

Maybe my story wasn't over.

Maybe, despite everything I had lost, I still had a chance to reclaim something.

I just had to start *fighting*.

At first, that fight was purely mental.

I was trapped in bed, unable to move at all.

But I started to *think* my way out.

I visualized walking, standing, and rebuilding myself from the inside out.

And then, little by little, my strength returned.

I don't know if it was because they had removed the psychotropic drugs clouding my mind or if the near-death experience actually rewired my brain.

Maybe it was both.

Either way, I now had a fierce determination to take my life back.

I knew I had to walk again.

I knew I had to talk again.

I knew I had to teach again.

And I was going to make it happen.

A Nightmare Within a Nightmare

Just as I was beginning to fight my way back, the world outside was burning down.

It was late summer of 2020, and California was engulfed in wildfires.

The sky turned a haunting, apocalyptic orange, the air thick with smoke and desperation.

And with each news report that reached me, my mind twisted the story into something even more terrifying.

Fires were creeping closer to my grandson's home in San Jose—just 15 miles away.

In my fragile state, I became convinced that I was going to die (for real, this time)—that we **all** were.

It wasn't a question of *if*, but *how*.

Would I starve to death if the staff abandoned the house to save themselves, leaving me trapped in my bed?

Would the flames consume everything, swallowing me whole before I could even take any more steps toward healing?

I had no control, no way out, no way to escape.

And the fear was suffocating.

When Fear Steals Your Last Bit of Strength

One night, panic overtook me.

I begged the caregivers to let me sleep on the floor, convinced that if the house filled with smoke, I could crawl beneath it and find some pocket of breathable air.

But they refused.

They had *never* let my feet touch the floor—not once for months—due to my history of falling.

Even as I grew stronger, even as I could have stood up on my own, they refused to let me try.

To them, my body was still fragile, my progress still invisible.

But to me?

I was being kept down on purpose.

And nothing was more infuriating than being forced to stay weak when I was finally ready to fight.

Abandoned, But Still Here

The wildfire chaos was bad enough, but the pandemic was still raging, and things inside Gwen's Place were falling apart, too.

One by one, I watched as her employees packed their things and left—until only one remained.

Enigmatic Tony.

Tony was now the only caregiver in the house.

He was responsible for everything—cooking, changing diapers, bathing, feeding.

His shifts stretched to 24 hours straight. Gwen stepped in for only a few hours here and there to give him a breather.

He rarely spoke and barely looked at me, moving like a machine on autopilot.

And so, I was left in near-total isolation, trapped in a house where everyone but Tony had walked away.

Even Gwen herself was struggling to keep things together.

At one point, only two residents remained—me and Gwen's own bedridden mother, who also suffered from **Lewy body dementia**.

The house became ever more so eerily silent.

No visitors.

No conversation.

Just the sound of my own thoughts clawing their way through the endless, empty hours.

And yet—despite it all—I was still here.

And I was still fighting.

The fires didn't take me.

The isolation didn't break me.

Somewhere deep inside, I could feel it—

The rewiring had already begun.

Crawling Back into My Life

The fires had eventually subsided, and with them, my panic.

154

But the fear had left its mark.

I had spent weeks convinced that death was closing in—whether from flames, starvation, or the slow, inevitable decline of my own mind.

And yet... I was still here.

Still alive.

Something inside me shifted again.

For the first time in a very long time, I wasn't just waiting to die—I was actively trying to survive.

But to do that, I had to start *moving*.

I had to stop waiting for permission to heal.

And so, I began my quiet rebellion.

Fortunately—or maybe miraculously—Gwen's Place lacked the alarms, barriers, and pressure pads that could have put an end to my nightly escapades. There were no shrill alerts blaring if my feet touched the ground, no restrictive devices confining me to my bed.

I was *free*, in the smallest, most fragile way.

And that freedom became my exhilarating lifeline.

Each stolen moment—each tiny rebellion—was a quiet victory, a whisper of the independence I had once known. Sneaking through the house, rediscovering movement, reclaiming my body—these were not just acts of survival; they were acts of defiance.

The world had written me off, but I was rewriting the ending.

In the stillness of those solitary hours, I found myself poring over my hospice notes and medication lists, determined to piece together the puzzle of what had happened to me.

Digging through transfer records in Gwen's office, I uncovered a detailed list of all the medications I had been prescribed before arriving here. The sheer number of them was staggering.

I wrote them all down carefully and methodically, knowing this information was vital.

It felt like assembling a puzzle in the dark—slow, uncertain, but empowering.

Each piece of knowledge was a step forward.

Each stolen moment, a quiet reclamation.

It wasn't much, but it was a start.

And from that start, I began to rebuild.

I had been given a mission—to help others.

But first?

I had to help *myself*.

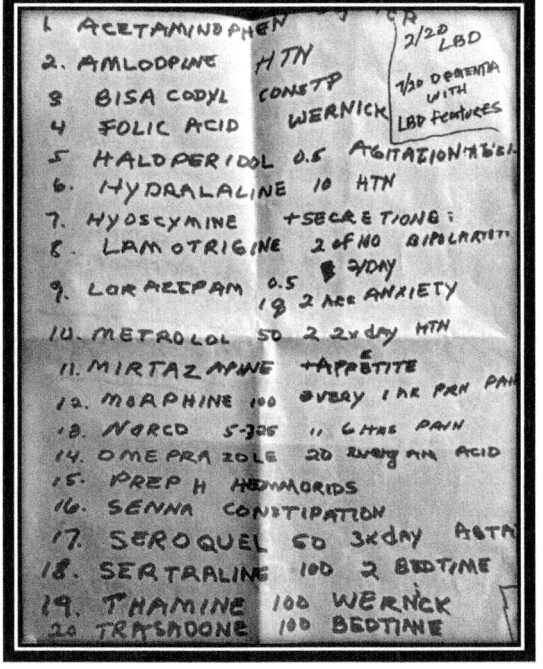

The End of Hospice

The world outside continued to crumble under COVID-19, yet inside Gwen's, my own crisis was shifting.

I was still here, but hospice?

Hospice had moved on.

Hospice care is meant to be re-evaluated and renewed regularly. Mine wasn't.

My certification wasn't extended, and just like that, I was no longer considered someone "actively dying."

Hospice had been a waiting room between life and death, and I had somehow walked out the wrong door.

I should have been relieved, but instead, I felt a new kind of panic.

Hospice had covered what little care I had left—a weekly nurse, a social worker who listened.

Without it, I would have nothing.

At one point, I even considered faking my decline, just to stay in the system.

But something inside me refused.

That ember of dignity—the same one that had kept me crawling back into life—it wouldn't let me pretend to be dying when I had worked so hard to survive.

So, instead of faking weakness, I embraced my slow and stubborn transformative journey.

My nurse noticed.

She began measuring my arms not for decline this time, but for progress.

I was gaining weight, regaining strength, and pulling myself back to life.

And oh, did my body come back with a *vengeance*.

The Hunger

My body had been starving for months—both physically and mentally.

And when my mind began to clear, something even stronger took over:

Hunger.

Not just the kind that gnawed at my stomach, but the kind that clawed at my soul.

The hunger to live again.

And so, I did something I hadn't done in ages—I ate.

I ate with reckless abandon, as if my body was trying to make up for lost time.

I became a midnight kitchen thief, creeping through the house like a feral creature, rediscovering the simple, visceral joy of being alive.

Nothing was off-limits.

Anything within reach was fair game.

Food tasted different; like every bite was infused with a second chance.

And for the first time in forever, I let myself savor it.

My grandson, Jeremy, had sent me a box of books and a bag of candy, a simple gift that became an unexpected lifeline to the outside world.

I rationed every piece of candy, allowing myself just one a day, treating each bite like a sacred ritual.

And then there were the books.

The first time I managed to read again, it was like returning to an old, familiar friend—one I hadn't realized I had lost.

Stephen King's *It* became my closest companion.

I clung to that book with a fierceness I couldn't explain, reading it not once, not twice, but *three* times.

Not just for entertainment—for **survival**.

The words became a tether to something bigger than my confined world.

They reminded me that life existed beyond these walls, beyond the silence, beyond the limitations my body had placed on me.

I was still here.

And I was **coming back**.

Facing the Invaluable Truth

Leaving hospice meant I had to face a new reality—one where I was technically not dying, but still not *free*.

The cost of staying off hospice was about $8,000 a month, and if you add all the 'extras,' that easily climbed to $10,000.

Financially, it was *crushing*.

But physically?

I was **winning**.

By late 2020, there was no denying it—I was coming back.

I could stand again. I could use a walker.

I could feed myself without assistance.

I could see the world beyond Gwen's Place in a way I hadn't in *so long*.

But what I didn't realize at the time was that my progress—slow and quiet as it was—was benefiting Gwen far more than it was benefiting me.

The stronger I became, the more I started to see the cracks in her carefully controlled version of reality.

If I could stand, if I could move, if I could care for myself, then why was I still here?

Why was she still insisting that I wasn't well enough to go home?

The truth crept in like an unwelcome guest—I had become more valuable to her as a paying resident than as a person regaining independence.

Gaslighting in the Guise of Care

Gwen spun a story—a dangerous, self-serving story.

She painted me as too weak, too confused, too far gone to leave. She whispered these lies to my family and friends, ensuring they never saw the real me—the me that was slowly but surely ready to reclaim my life.

And I believed her, *too*.

I was being gaslit, though I didn't recognize it at the time.

She and Tony *constantly* told me I was too sick to be up and moving around, and in my already fragile state, I didn't push back.

Even when they refused to let me practice walking during the day.

Even when they panicked if I so much as shifted my weight.

Even when they punished me for trying.

They claimed it was all about "safety and licensure," but my emotional well-being? That was an afterthought.

The mere act of trying to stand would send them into a frenzy, met with sharp reprimands and thinly veiled threats.

If I tested my own strength, they'd dangle what little freedom I had finally earned over my head—

- Taking away my TV time
- Revoking my control of the remote
- Shutting my door completely at night

They *knew* that a closed door made me feel like a prisoner locked in a cell.

And they used it *anyway*.

The message was clear: Stay down. Stay silent. Stay powerless.

And so, I did... *sort of*.

I kept my progress to myself, retreating into a quiet defiance, determined to continue reclaiming my independence in secret.

The Call That Changed Everything

My slow improvement and the staggering expense of staying off hospice—likely compounded by the reverse mortgage situation—made staying at Gwen's unsustainable.

The reverse mortgage rules about nursing home stays, which limited my time to one year, had already forced multiple failed trials at home before I ended up here.

And then, after nearly a year of "confinement" at Gwen's, Ty called with a bombshell:

"You're coming home in three weeks."

I was **stunned**.

At that point, even though I had secretly begun walking without Gwen's knowledge, feeding and diapering myself, and clearing mentally without hallucinations, I still felt utterly powerless.

I had convinced myself that going home was impossible.

I believed I was doomed to remain at Gwen's—or some other confining facility—forever. That only a *miracle* could possibly send me back home.

I had long since given up hope.

Since my admission to Gwen's and the onset of COVID, no family member had offered any words of encouragement about the possibility of returning home.

The lack of control over my life, the trauma of repeated failures, and the weight of isolation had left me gutted.

I stopped asking to come home long ago.

I resigned myself to the belief that I didn't deserve anything more than existing in this room.

And then—those beautiful, simple words:

"You're coming home."

That changed **everything**.

Suddenly, what had once felt impossible became *real*.

For the first time in what seemed like forever, I began to envision life beyond Gwen's Place.

The idea of coming home didn't just signify a change of scenery—

It promised a chance to fulfill my mission of **reclaiming my life**.

CHAPTER 23: MY PERSONAL "AFTERLIFE"

Despite my growing determination to regain my strength, there was a time—somewhere around the eighth or ninth month at Gwen's—when I had to hide my progress.

I kept my ability to walk a secret, afraid of what might happen if they knew just how much I had improved. Was I protecting myself? Or was I just afraid that if they saw me standing, they'd find a way to knock me back down?

Gwen, for all her warmth and charisma, had her own struggles—her mother, confined to her room, bedridden, silent, slipping deeper into Lewy body dementia. Watching me regain what her mother had permanently lost must have been heartbreaking.

By the time I walked out the door on February 17, 2021, Gwen's Place had dwindled to just one other patient. Not long after, it shut down for good—a casualty of COVID-era financial collapse, another fragment of the crumbling care system.

I should have felt nothing but relief as I left. And yet, there was something unnerving about stepping outside.

Maybe it was because, despite months of frustration, I had developed something dangerously close to Stockholm syndrome.

I liked Gwen—she was kind, beautiful, and extremely charismatic—I understood her. I had empathized with the people who held me back—who convinced me, in some twisted way, that I was safer here, caged but cared for, rather than free and failing.

And then, just as I was about to escape into my newfound freedom—

Gwen dropped a bombshell.

"Oh," she said casually as if we were discussing the weather. "I've known for a while now that you could use the walker pretty well."

I stopped. Stared.

She had *known*.

For how long?

And yet, for months, she had still painted me as too fragile, too impaired, too much of a fall risk.

Why?

Had she done it out of concern? Maybe.

Had she done it because keeping me there meant keeping her facility open? Probably.

Had I unknowingly been a VIP client in a place on the verge of collapse? Without a doubt.

I could have been angry, but mostly, I just felt tired.

Desperation does strange things to people. And, in the end, I was just another casualty of a broken system—a system that convinces people to trade autonomy for safety and then strips them of both.

But as I 'walked' out the door that day, walker in hand, one thing was undeniable:

I felt *free*.

It's What You Don't See That Hurts Most

Stepping back into my condo after nearly a year away should have felt like a triumphant homecoming.

Instead, it felt like walking onto a Broadway stage that had been stripped of its set.

Ty and Tanya had worked tirelessly to make my home safer for me—but in doing so, they had also erased everything that made it mine.

My gorgeous leather couch was gone. The revolving recliner that had once wrapped me in comfort had vanished.

The once-grand, wooden entertainment center that had anchored my living room had been ripped from the wall, leaving behind gaping holes.

And my lovely fish tank? Replaced by emptiness, as if my living room had been subjected to a furniture apocalypse.

It wasn't just aesthetic changes. It was a complete overhaul of my existence.

Independence, Revoked

The next thing I noticed was that *everything* I had previously been using to connect with the outside world had also been removed.

My cell phone was nowhere to be found.

My specialized PAC Bell phone, the one that converted voice messages into text—a lifeline for someone like me? Erased.

My ID, credit cards, and any access to money? Gone.

I had no way to call, text, or even order pizza in a moment of rebellion.

And the TV? Off-limits.

The remote wasn't mine to touch anymore.

Making my own coffee? Nope.

Fixing my own food? Forbidden.

Riding the handicapped bus system I had relied on before? Absolutely not.

And driving? Well, that had been out of the picture for years, but now it was as if my entire existence was being placed under guardianship.

The unspoken message was clear:

If it involved buttons, wheels, or hot liquids, it wasn't for me.

I wasn't returning *home*.

I was returning to another version of Gwen's, where I still had no control over my *life*.

I had spent months trying to prove to myself that I could still function.

And now, I wasn't even trusted to turn on my own damn television.

Looks Like a Natural Disaster Came Through Here

Walking around in my condo felt like stepping into the aftermath of a highly selective tornado—one that had surgically targeted my personal belongings with ruthless efficiency.

But it wasn't just my *belongings* that had been stripped away.

It was the *essence* of who I was.

My shoes were nearly wiped out.

My jewelry had been crammed into a single, pitifully small box.

My extensive earring collection—roughly 50 mismatched pairs that had been a signature of my personality—was completely decimated.

Aside from my cherished collections of Dickens' Village houses and pewter horses, nearly everything had vanished. Even the little things—my makeup, towels, and wall art—were gone, replaced by a stark, utilitarian version of my former life.

I had spent months wondering if I would ever come back to myself.

And now that I was here...

It felt like there was nothing left of me to return to.

My beautiful little fenced yard, once bursting with flowers and life, had withered into a tangle of neglect—an overgrown reminder of all the time I had lost.

Even my old bedroom was no longer mine.

Ty had turned it into his home office, his desk now residing where my old life had been.

I understood. I truly did.

He and Tanya had prepared for a version of me that never came home— either because I didn't make it or where I was permanently held "in custody" (a term that felt all too fitting).

But understanding it didn't make it hurt less.

My condo had become a controlled environment, designed for safety but stripped of self-expression.

And I was now a guest in my own life.

Still a Prison Cell, Just with Better Furniture

The disillusionment didn't stop at the stripped-down condo or the missing pieces of my old life. No, front and center, like a morbid centerpiece, was a hospital bed in the middle of my once-cozy living room.

Flanking it was a stiff recliner—the kind that's built for function, not comfort—and a wheelchair that loomed like a permanent fixture of my future.

The big TV—once something I could navigate effortlessly—was now controlled through an unnecessarily convoluted system. And, as if that weren't frustrating enough, I was informed—in the kind of gentle yet firm tone usually reserved for toddlers—that I would "*never* be trusted" with the remote again.

At first, it was strictly off-limits.

But before long, I started tinkering with it in secret, and little by little, the familiarity crept back until, almost without realizing it, I had relearned how to use it all over again.

Meals on Wheels had been ordered, and while I dearly missed Tanya's home-cooked meals, I bit my tongue and swallowed my pride because I knew it would relieve some of her burden.

And, in my zeal to be thought of as a completely independent woman again, I rehearsed and polished a narrative for the Meals on Wheels representative—appearances *do* matter, after all.

(For the record, I am very grateful for the service. It gives Tanya a much-needed break, and that alone makes it worth enduring the occasional mystery casserole.)

But then, there was the pièce de résistance of my new reality:

A nanny cam system linked to an Alexa digital assistant—a setup that transformed my entire existence into a low-budget reality show.

Minus the paycheck. Minus the glamour.

And definitely minus the option to vote anyone off the island.

Mirror, Mirror, What the Hell Happened?

The *real* shocker came when I finally caught a glimpse of myself in the mirror.

(Fun fact: long-term care facilities often remove or cover mirrors because they can distress residents experiencing delusions. Turns out, that's not a bad strategy.)

Because what I saw was **not** me.

Staring back was a very skinny old woman, her gray-streaked, oily hair limp, her skin discolored, her frame so thin it looked like it had been whittled down by time itself.

And the chin whiskers—dear God.

I had enough to rival a goat in the Swiss Alps.

Someone once called wrinkles "wise cracks," but mine looked more like the extended family of the Grand Canyon.

And then there were the skin barnacles—a delightful term used by dermatologists that only adds insult to injury.

I had enough of them to qualify for a starring role in *Pirates of the Caribbean.*

It was not a good look.

But over time, with a little stealth grooming, things improved.

My skin cleared up.

The goat whiskers were eliminated—shoutout to the friend who smuggled in a pair of tweezers like we were in some kind of underground beauty contraband ring.

My shoulder-length hair, once an oily mess, evolved into a fashionably silver-streaked style.

I may be an octogenarian, but I'd like to think I've turned into a rather cute one.

Just don't ask what I'm up to with those tweezers in the one corner of the bathroom the nanny cam doesn't reach.

Some secrets are best kept unsupervised.

What a Witch

For a time, I still wore diapers at night—a humiliating necessity based on Gwen's advice.

Which meant, at times, Ty had to change them.

I don't think I need to spell out how awful that was for both of us.

On top of that, they had been told I needed help showering, even though Tony had already let me handle it on my own back at Gwen's.

Apparently, Gwen had told Tanya I wasn't safe to shower alone—likely to ensure that my family didn't think I was ready to leave her care.

And it worked.

My family also didn't know that they could have requested a **physical therapy (PT)** or **occupational therapy (OT) evaluation** for me upon returning home—an oversight that, in hindsight, could have changed everything.

Gwen had convinced them that I was barely mobile, wheelchair-bound, and incapable of independence.

And because they trusted her word, they never knew about the resources that could have helped them navigate my return home in a way that wasn't so overwhelming.

This—***this right here***—is one of the biggest reasons I am writing this book.

Because caregivers deserve to know the options available to them.

They deserve to know what support exists, what rights they have, and how to make informed choices without being manipulated by a broken system.

Maybe, if my family had known, the hostility that developed between Tanya and me might have been avoided.

Maybe she wouldn't have been so exhausted.

Maybe I wouldn't have been such an absolute nightmare.

Because let's be real—I ***was*** a nightmare.

Here was Tanya, my daughter-in-law, giving up her time, her energy, and, frankly, her patience to help me with bathing, hygiene, and basic care.

And how did I repay her?

By being an absolute ***witch***.

It's humbling—and honestly, embarrassing—to admit.

But if telling this truth can help another caregiver avoid the pain Tanya endured, then maybe this book will have done its job.

Two Steps Forward, One Step Back

About three months after returning home, something incredible started happening.

At first, it was just fleeting moments of complete clarity—like brief flickers of light in a dark tunnel.

But then, those flickers grew stronger.

My mind—once a foggy, tangled mess of confusion—was sharpening.

It was as if someone had hit the rewind button on my brain, slowly reversing the cognitive decline that had gripped me for over twelve years.

Memories I thought were lost forever began resurfacing.

Thoughts felt clearer. Words came easier.

I was waking up—not just in body, but in mind and spirit.

It felt like my brain was repairing itself, little by little, as though it had simply been waiting for the right conditions to heal.

Maybe it was neuroplasticity at work.

Maybe it was somatic healing—my body and mind finally syncing again.

Or maybe, just maybe, it was something bigger.

But just as my mind was coming back online, my body decided to stage a rebellion.

The Pain No One Believed

At first, it was just a dull ache.

Then, the stomach pain became unbearable.

I couldn't eat.

I cried constantly.

And then came the vomiting—violent, unrelenting, leaving me weak and drained of every ounce of progress I had fought for.

Ty and Tanya, already exhausted from months of caregiving, assumed it was just another phase of my decline.

They suggested that perhaps I wasn't "wiping myself" properly—a suspicion that left me drowning in guilt.

And when I continued to grow sicker, their frustration turned into doubt.

They believed I was exaggerating for attention; an assumption Gwen had planted in their minds long before I ever returned home.

I had seen it happen before—to countless patients in my years as an SLP.

When someone lives in a haze of cognitive dysfunction long enough, their words—even when true—begin to lose credibility.

And now, here I was, screaming in pain, yet no one was listening.

Three agonizing days passed.

Then, finally, Ty took me to the ER.

And there, doctors discovered the truth:

A baseball-sized tumor.

Immediate surgery was required.

Thankfully, it wasn't cancer—but those two weeks of waiting for the biopsy results felt like an eternity.

Yet, in a strange way, the hospital stay was almost... enjoyable.

People cared for me there.

They treated me with kindness.

I had visitors—including an old classmate and fellow SLP, someone who saw me as I was, not as the broken thing I had become.

The contrast was stark—at home, I had felt like an inconvenience, an obligation, a problem to be managed.

But here?

Here, I was just a person who needed care, and they gave it freely.

The Short-Sleeve Battle

Back home, everything felt different—and not in the way I had hoped.

In an effort to cheer me up, Tanya had bought me some cute new clothes.

It was a thoughtful gesture, but when a visitor stopped by, I was handed a short-sleeved shirt to wear.

A shirt that left my painfully thin, sagging arms completely exposed.

A harsh, unforgiving reminder of the 100 pounds I had lost.

I begged—actually *begged*—for long sleeves.

It sounds trivial, I know.

But it wasn't about the fabric.

It was about dignity.

It was about control over my own body.

I just wanted one small victory—a sliver of autonomy in a life that had been dictated by others for far too long.

But my request was denied.

And in that moment, I felt as powerless as I had when I was trapped at Gwen's.

Because it wasn't just about a shirt.

It was about the constant, crushing realization that my choices weren't mine anymore.

That my comfort—my preferences, my autonomy—didn't matter.

And this wasn't the first time clothing had shaken me to my core.

Years earlier, I had struggled to pull on a simple muumuu—my mind and body so uncooperative that I had to call my housekeeper for help.

That moment had hit me like a brick wall—the first time I truly understood how far I had slipped.

But now? Now, I have a new memory.

A *better* one.

I still remember the sheer triumph of putting on my nightgown without assistance—no housekeeper, no helper, just me.

It wasn't just an article of clothing.

It was proof. Proof that I was coming back.

Proof that I was regaining what dementia had tried to steal from me.

Wrestling with Independence

Showering was another battleground—one that was about more than just hygiene.

At first, Tanya had to bathe me entirely. I hated it.

Not because of her—but because of what it meant.

It meant I was helpless. It meant I had lost control over my own body.

It meant dementia had stolen yet another piece of my dignity.

I yelled, "F*ck!" and started crying. I wasn't cursing at her—but at myself.

But Tanya didn't see the deeper pain. She mistook my outburst as *anger*—as if I were lashing out at her instead of the situation.

And in my desperation, I begged for the chance to shower myself—to prove that I wasn't as broken as I felt.

Tanya, rightfully cautious, wasn't sure I was ready.

In her mind, I had been bedbound for so long that I needed to relearn how to do even the most basic things—like standing in the shower without falling.

But that logic didn't make it any easier.

It didn't lessen the sting of being treated like a fragile thing—a person too weak, too dependent, too much of a risk to be trusted with her own care.

And so, as my strength returned, so did my defiance.

The Not-So-Great Escape

The frustration had been building for weeks.

I was gaining back pieces of myself, yet I still felt trapped, still felt like they saw me as a patient—not as a person coming back to life.

And then, the last straw—I thought Ty and Tanya were taking away my TV remote.

My only connection to the world. My last shred of control.

Something inside me snapped. I decided I was leaving.

So, I did.

I grabbed my walker, shuffled out the door in my pajamas, and set off into the world—because damn it, if I couldn't have my remote, I was going to find *someone* who would listen to me.

Someone who would take me to social services.

Now, imagine it: an elderly woman, hair wild, eyes blazing with righteous indignation, determinedly hobbling down the streets of San Mateo like a fugitive from a nursing home.

I must have been quite the sight.

The first person I encountered was the gardener.

He looked startled—and then promptly retreated, as if he wanted no part of whatever rebellion I was staging.

Then came a woman walking her dog.

She gave me a look of pity so profound that it still lingers in my memory—like she had just witnessed a tragic spectacle, something she wasn't sure if she should intervene in or simply walk away from.

Before I could get very far, Ty found me.

He didn't yell. He didn't scold me.

He just gently took me home—where I sulked like a grounded teenager.

The Helicopter Caregivers

Later, Ty helped me see the situation from Tanya's perspective.

Her rules, her hypervigilance—they weren't about *controlling* me.

They were about *protecting* me.

She worried about my UTIs, knowing they could lead to delusions and medical crises.

She worried about me falling—about one bad accident setting me back months, or worse, undoing everything I had fought to regain.

And I was blind to all of it.

All I saw was someone stripping away my independence.

What she saw was someone she was desperately trying to keep safe.

Looking back, I can see how our opposing needs clashed like two colliding storms.

I was fighting to prove I could take care of myself.

She was fighting to make sure I never had to go through another emergency again.

We both needed understanding.

We both needed grace.

But at the time, all we could see was frustration and exhaustion.

And to make matters worse, Gwen had fed my family false information before I ever got home.

She had made me sound far more helpless than I was, leading Ty and Tanya to believe that I was still on the brink of disaster.

So, when I pushed back against their help, it felt like an insult to all they had sacrificed to care for me.

They thought I was ungrateful.

I thought they were overbearing.

None of us saw that the truth was buried somewhere in between.

Mea Culpa

Back before dementia stole my independence, before my health collapsed, I had spent years mentoring students—teaching them the art of communication, the importance of careful language, the power of words.

And yet, in one of the most critical moments of my life, I forgot all of it.

I forgot that words can heal, but they can also cut deep.

Years earlier, two of my Chinese students in Project Read had taught me that, in their culture, brutal honesty is not only acceptable, it's *honored*.

Unfortunately, I had taken that lesson and wielded it like a sword.

I lashed out.

At Tanya. At Ty.

At the very people who had given up so much to care for me.

I was so desperate to reclaim my independence that I didn't see how my words were hurting the people I loved most.

By the time I realized the damage I had done, it was too late to take back the things I had said.

But I could try to make amends.

I could try to fix what I had broken.

So, after my dramatic (and failed) escape attempt, I did the only thing I could.

I apologized.

Not just once. Not just casually.

But over and over, in every way I knew how.

But here's the thing about seeking forgiveness—sometimes, the hardest part isn't getting others to forgive you.

Sometimes, the hardest part is forgiving yourself.

Because no matter how many apologies I gave...

No matter how many ways I tried to make it right...

That inner voice still whispered:

"It's all my fault."

And if I was ever going to truly move forward, I had to find a way to silence that voice—or at the very least, learn how to live with it.

A Nanny Cam Revelation

Years later, during a long overdue visit, Tanya and I had a revealing conversation—one that finally explained a few of the lingering mysteries of my early days back home.

She admitted that, for a while, she had been directing Ty's actions through the nanny cam.

Yes, that's right.

My every move—every attempt at sneaking a cookie, every minor rebellion—had been under surveillance. If I got up, she'd know. If I so much as rustled my bedsheets suspiciously, she could rewind and investigate.

At the time, it felt like an outright invasion of privacy—*Big Sister Is Watching You*—but looking back, I can see that it was never about control. It was about *concern*. My health had been fragile, my body unpredictable, and they were trying to prevent a fall that could land me right back in the place we all feared most: another facility.

These days, the nanny cam has been adjusted to be less intrusive. Now, it only triggers an alert for loud noises (like a fall) or clear distress signals (such as yelling or a desperate plea for help). Which, let's be honest, is an improvement—I no longer feel like a reality TV contestant being monitored for dramatic effect.

But, of course, there were *other* moments that tested my patience—and theirs.

Take, for example, the time Ty grabbed my phone, convinced I was texting something negative about them. Now, to be fair, I *wasn't* (at least, not that time). But I won't pretend I was an angel. I had my guilty little habits—sneaking treats, strategically dumping food I didn't like, and, yes, occasionally being difficult for sport.

Still, for every act of quiet defiance, there was an equal and opposite wave of remorse. Because, despite my stubborn streak, I wanted to make things right.

From Contrition to Confidence

These days, my focus is on building a better relationship with Tanya and Ty—not just as caregivers but as family.

I genuinely appreciate everything they've done for me, and I recognize just how much I still rely on them. But at the same time, I'm working to reclaim more of my independence—one small victory at a time.

Each step forward—whether it's handling my own meals, regaining control of my own schedule, or simply proving that I'm capable—lightens their burden and reconnects me with the person I used to be.

This entire experience has been a lesson in patience—for all of us.

I've realized that my desperate attempts to reclaim control sometimes veered into outright rebellion, while their instinct to protect me sometimes crossed into overprotection. We were all learning, struggling, and navigating a situation none of us had ever been trained for.

But through it all, I've gained something unexpected: a deeper appreciation for what they endured and the sacrifices they made.

And, perhaps most importantly, I've come to understand that true independence isn't just about doing everything on your own.

It's about knowing when to lean on others—

And when to let them lean on you.

And Now, Some Reflection

Caregiving—whether by family, friends, or professionals—is nothing short of a rollercoaster ride with a broken safety bar. It's a relentless loop of compassion, exhaustion, frustration, guilt, and love, sometimes all at once. The sheer emotional weight of it can push even the most patient souls to their limits.

Looking back on my own journey, I can only hope that those who were by my side—who bore the brunt of my worst moments—can see the truth: what they once called my 'loathsome behaviors' weren't intentional acts of selfishness or cruelty. They were symptoms of a brain in crisis, the collision of genetics, disease, and trauma playing out in real time.

I have *always* tried to be a good person. And I continue to try—practicing compassion not just for others but also, finally, for myself. I strive to lead a life of meaning, one guided by intention rather than regret.

And here's the thing: four years later, I've made it.

Against all odds, my quality of life has drastically improved. I am far more independent, and while my journey wasn't easy on my family, Ty and Tanya's support has remained unwavering. They still provide supplies, manage paperwork, bring treats, and fill my never-ending pill container. Their help has been invaluable, though I know the price they've paid has been steep.

Caregiving is often described as "thankless," but that word doesn't quite capture the full picture. It's a role that devours time, energy, and sometimes even health itself. Studies show that caregivers are at higher risk for chronic illness, reduced productivity, and even premature death due to prolonged emotional and physical strain. When I lashed out, when I was lost in delusions, when my behavior tested every last ounce of their patience, I know now that detachment might have been their only way to survive it.

Still, even with the weight they've carried, they've never abandoned me.

Ty and Tanya continue to support me as Family and Medical Leave caregivers, and I remain under palliative care through Kaiser. My safety is enhanced by an Alexa device that acts as a digital watchdog, and I've embraced my growing autonomy rather than resenting the precautions around me. I've also come to deeply appreciate the lifestyle changes they implemented—because, as it turns out, they may have done far more for my turnaround than any doctor ever did.

Recent research suggests that a high percentage of disease modification stems from behavioral and environmental shifts—so much so that they can even influence **DNA plasticity** (the idea that your DNA isn't totally fixed or set in stone—it can adapt or change how it works based on your environment, lifestyle, or experiences). In other words, while science races to develop cures for neurodegenerative conditions, the choices we make each day—our routines, our stress levels, our interactions with the world—are already shaping the outcomes of our health.

Finding Balance in a New Life

Though some frustrations linger and old wounds from my dementia-like behavior haven't fully healed, one thing remains unwavering: my deep love and respect for my son.

I am profoundly proud to be his mother. He now works as a medical actuary—a role that requires not only advanced training in mathematics and statistics but also a sharp understanding of healthcare trends, risk analysis, and long-term outcome modeling. Becoming an actuary isn't for the faint of heart; it takes years of rigorous exams, specialized coursework, and a mind built for solving the kinds of complex problems most of us run from. That's my Ty.

And while I admire his brilliance, I also understand the flip side of it. His fear—his caution, his instinct to control what he can—comes from a place rooted in logic *and* love. As someone who evaluates risk for a living, how could he not ask the hardest question of all: *"What if it happens again?"* What if everything I've regained slips away?

It's a fear I wish I could erase for him. But I know why it lingers. When you've walked through the fire, you don't forget the heat.

Still, for now, my life feels more balanced and stable. I've found ways to stay connected—to people, to purpose, and, most importantly, to myself.

I now have a Senior Peer volunteer counselor who visits weekly—a role I once filled for others before my decline.

I can use the TV remote without frustration (a small but mighty victory).

Earlier, when my mind was still in flux, I attempted a Zoom-captioned support group through Peninsula Family Service, but it wasn't the right fit. Then, I joined a Friendly Visitors program (www.friendlyvoices.org), where I have weekly calls with a volunteer, something that provides genuine comfort and connection.

But perhaps the most important constant in my transformative journey has been writing.

It keeps me tethered to both my past and my future.

My days are now filled with meaningful activities—light housekeeping, preparing my own meals, reading voraciously (as if trying to make up for lost time), and contributing to humor sites (because if I don't laugh at some of this, what's the alternative?).

I even continue my relentless deep dive into neurodegenerative research, a fascination that keeps my brain engaged and reminds me of the very science that may have saved me.

In Remission—Or Something More?

Astonishingly, the dementia-like features that once defined my life have disappeared entirely.

Not just remission. Gone.

My doctors at Kaiser remain baffled. My latest MRI showed only minimal brain shrinkage and mild encephalopathy—nothing out of the ordinary for someone my age. My word-finding issues and minor executive function deficits are manageable. The insomnia, occasional tremors, and body aches persist, but cortisone injections and a recent hip replacement have left me nearly pain-free.

More importantly, I am no longer manic.

I am no longer depressed, disoriented, or afraid.

Instead, I am humbled.

Humbled by the love and care that carried me through. Humbled by the incredible, inexplicable turnaround that medicine still can't fully explain.

For the first time in a long time, I truly value my life—perhaps more than I ever have before.

The Ultimate Question: How?

So, here's the question that still lingers—how did I go from being mere hours away from death, confined to a hospice bed, to this?

How did I move from the brink of oblivion to a life of independence, curiosity, and purpose?

Was it science? Neuroplasticity rewiring my brain in ways we don't fully understand? A shift in brain chemistry that medicine has yet to define?

Or was it something beyond explanation?

Divine intervention? Fate? A sheer, stubborn refusal to let dementia have the last laugh?

Maybe it was all of the above.

Or maybe my story is simply the medical equivalent of a plot twist no one saw coming.

Whatever the answer, the journey to uncover the truth starts *now*.

CHAPTER 24: DEFINING MY DEMENTIAS

Before we can begin to dissect the mystery of my survival, it's crucial to first understand the monsters I was battling—two formidable neurodegenerative diseases that *don't just fade away.*

Lewy Body Dementia: The Ultimate Deceiver

Lewy body dementia (LBD) is the chameleon of neurodegenerative diseases. It mimics Alzheimer's, Parkinson's, and psychiatric disorders so convincingly that even seasoned neurologists often miss it.

It is caused by the accumulation of Lewy bodies—abnormal protein deposits of **alpha-synuclein**—in the nerve cells of the brain. These unwelcome intruders disrupt cognitive function, movement, sleep, and autonomic regulation. And because the symptoms ebb and flow, appearing and disappearing like a cruel trickster, LBD often leaves both patients and doctors questioning their own reality.

Despite being the second most common degenerative dementia after Alzheimer's, LBD remains alarmingly underdiagnosed. In fact, many people diagnosed with Alzheimer's or Parkinson's are only discovered posthumously to have had LBD all along (*10 Things You Should Know About LBD – Lewy Body Dementia Association*, n.d.).

The Two Faces of Lewy Body Dementia

LBD presents in two primary forms:

- Dementia with Lewy bodies (DLB): Starts with cognitive issues—hallucinations, attention deficits, and fluctuating alertness—before motor symptoms appear.

- **Parkinson's disease dementia (PDD):** Begins with movement problems typical of Parkinson's—**tremors, rigidity, and muscle stiffness**—with cognitive decline emerging much later.

While these two conditions seem distinct, they share the same underlying pathology. The distinction is mostly about which symptoms show up first.

LBD's Shape-Shifting Symptoms

LBD isn't just one disease—it's *many* diseases in one. It has an entire arsenal of symptoms that appear and disappear unpredictably, making it one of the most baffling and frustrating neurological disorders (*10 Things You Should Know About LBD,* n.d.):

- **Cognitive Impairments:** Unlike Alzheimer's, memory loss isn't always the main issue. Instead, people struggle with **fluctuating cognition, visual-spatial difficulties,** and **executive function deficits.** A person might seem perfectly normal in the morning and completely lost by afternoon.

- Motor Symptoms: LBD has Parkinsonism features—tremors, muscle rigidity, bradykinesia (slow movement), and postural instability—making movement difficult.

- **Sleep Disorders:** Many with LBD experience **REM sleep behavior disorder (RBD),** acting out their dreams, sometimes violently.

- Autonomic Dysfunction: LBD disrupts the autonomic nervous system, causing wild blood pressure fluctuations, dizziness, urinary problems, constipation, and difficulty regulating body temperature.

- Neuropsychiatric Symptoms: Depression, anxiety, paranoia, hallucinations (especially vivid visual ones), delusions, and mood swings are common.

Little-Known LBD Facts That Caregivers Should Know

Because of LBD's erratic nature, many families and caregivers discover the hard way just how unpredictable and challenging this disease can be:

- **Extreme Sensitivity to Medications:** Traditional antipsychotic drugs (like **Haldol** and **Risperidone**) can cause severe reactions, worsening symptoms, or even sudden death. Patients with LBD may experience severe **sedation**, **immobility**, or dangerous **drops in blood pressure** when given these medications. Always consult with a specialist before trying any psychiatric drugs (*10 Things You Should Know About LBD*, n.d.).

- **Cognition Can Change Hourly:** Unlike Alzheimer's, where cognitive decline is steady, LBD patients can fluctuate dramatically. One moment, they might seem fully present, and the next, they can't recognize their own home (LaChappelle, 2024).

- **Hallucinations Can Be Vivid and Bizarre:** LBD patients often see highly detailed people, animals, or creatures. Some find comfort in their visions, like seeing deceased loved ones, while others are terrorized by shadowy figures that feel all too real (LaChappelle, 2024).

- **Sudden Falls Are a Red Flag:** Many LBD patients fall years before they are diagnosed, often due to autonomic instability, balance issues, or muscle freezing (*What Is Lewy Body Dementia? Causes, Symptoms, and Treatments*, 2021).

- **Sleep Disorders Can Appear Decades Before Diagnosis:** REM sleep behavior disorder—where people physically act out their dreams—can precede cognitive symptoms by 10 to 20 years (*What Is Lewy Body Dementia? Causes, Symptoms, and Treatments*, 2021).

Diagnosing the Undiagnosable

LBD is routinely misdiagnosed. Many patients are initially told they have Alzheimer's, Parkinson's, or even a psychiatric disorder. Diagnosing LBD requires a combination of neurological exams, cognitive testing, sleep studies, and brain imaging (Loeb & Loeb, 2020).

While there is no cure, treatments focus on managing symptoms:

- **Medications:** Cholinesterase inhibitors (like **Donepezil**) can help with cognitive symptoms, while **Levodopa** may assist with motor function (*What Is Lewy Body Dementia? Causes, Symptoms, and Treatments*, 2021).

- **Therapies: Physical, occupational, and speech therapy** can help maintain independence (LaChappelle, 2024).

- **Lifestyle Adjustments:** Minimizing stress, maintaining structure, and avoiding medication pitfalls are critical. A simple infection or medication change can send an LBD patient into sudden, severe decline (LaChappelle, 2024).

Frontotemporal Dementia: The Rogue Villain

While I was also given a presumptive diagnosis of **Frontotemporal Dementia (FTD)** back in 2018, my symptoms leaned much more heavily toward LBD. However, because FTD presents very differently than other dementias, it's worth understanding.

FTD is caused by the progressive degeneration of the frontal and temporal lobes of the brain. Unlike Alzheimer's or LBD, memory loss isn't the primary issue. Instead, behavioral and language changes take center stage. This is why FTD is often mistaken for a psychiatric disorder (*What Are Frontotemporal Disorders? Causes, Symptoms, and Treatment*, 2021).

Signs of FTD Include:

- **Drastic personality shifts**—people become impulsive, rude, or inappropriate.

- **Compulsive or repetitive behaviors**—hoarding, overeating, touching objects repeatedly.

- **Loss of empathy and emotional blunting**—difficulty recognizing others' emotions.

- **Speech and language difficulties**—aphasia, trouble with grammar, or speaking in gibberish.

How LBD and FTD Are Different

- LBD patients hallucinate; FTD patients usually do not.

- FTD patients lose social filters early and may act inappropriately.

- LBD fluctuates (good days and bad days); FTD is steadily progressive.

Bringing it All Together

Understanding these two dementias is essential because they shaped my journey up to and back from the edge of death's door.

At my worst, I had 30 out of 34 LBD markers—including hallucinations, aphasia, tremors, delusions, drooling, paranoia, insomnia, and all facets of cognitive decline.

And yet... I got better.

So, what happened?

That's exactly what we'll explore next.

CHAPTER 25: CHASING CLUES TO MY COMEBACK

Looking back, it's impossible to pinpoint a single reason for my astonishing—some might say impossible—return from the brink of death.

I've spent years wrestling with different possibilities, sifting through science, medicine, and my own lived experience in an attempt to make sense of what defied all expectations.

At my lowest, I was bedbound, hallucinating, incapable of feeding myself, and declared beyond hope. The medical community had essentially stamped my file with an expiration date.

And yet, against all odds, here I am. But how?

The Puzzle with Many Pieces

I honestly do not believe there is one single answer. Instead, what happened was likely the result of a complex interplay of neurological, genetic, psychological, and even spiritual factors. Some pieces of the puzzle fit neatly into medical explanations, while others remain shrouded in mystery.

But if we're going to attempt to untangle the how and why of my return from the brink, we have to start somewhere. And one of the biggest suspects? The pharmaceutical rollercoaster I had been trapped on for years.

1. Medication Overload and Sudden Withdrawal

For most of my adult life, I had been prescribed medication after medication, each one added on top of the last, until my daily routine resembled something closer to a science experiment than actual healthcare. At times, I was juggling more than 10 different prescriptions—antipsychotics, mood stabilizers, sedatives, and many other over-the-counter remedies meant to keep me "stable."

Instead of feeling better, I felt foggy, exhausted, and increasingly detached from reality. But that's just the cost of treating neurological conditions, right?

Then, hospice happened.

Nearly all of my medications—which numbered **20** at the time—were stripped away overnight. Hospice doesn't aim to cure—it focuses on comfort. And in their eyes, I was beyond saving.

No more psychotropics. No more mood stabilizers. No more medications masking my symptoms while possibly making them worse.

While for most people, suddenly stopping multiple medications would be a recipe for disaster (and in some cases, even fatal), for me, it may have been the exact shock my system needed. Without the constant bombardment of pharmaceuticals, my brain finally had a chance to reset.

Could it be that my so-called dementia was being exacerbated—or even outright caused—by the very medications meant to help me?

The Perils of Polypharmacy: When More Isn't Always Better

Polypharmacy—taking multiple medications at once—is common among older adults. In some cases, it's necessary. But it's also a well-documented risk factor for cognitive impairment, increased falls, and adverse drug reactions.

Research has linked polypharmacy to **mild cognitive impairment** (MCI) and even full-blown dementia in the elderly (Chippa & Roy, 2023), raising an unsettling possibility:

What if my symptoms weren't just the result of a degenerative disease? What if they were being chemically induced?

One particularly eye-opening case study found that psychiatric polypharmacy can lead to specific cognitive dysfunction. The real kicker? Patients who stopped taking psychiatric medications showed cognitive improvement (Valtonen & Karrasch, 2020).

For years, I had been on a cocktail of medications that were known to sedate, dull, and even impair cognitive function. I had accepted the side effects as a necessary trade-off for stability. But what if I had been medicated into cognitive decline?

Deprescribing: Sometimes Less is More

The concept of **deprescribing**—carefully tapering off unnecessary medications—has gained recognition as a powerful intervention for improving cognitive function in older adults.

The National Institute on Aging warns that unnecessary medications increase the risk of cognitive decline and that reducing medication load could actually help prevent further deterioration (National Institute on Aging, 2021).

But before anyone rushes to throw Grandma's pills in the trash, let's be clear:

Deprescribing must ***always*** be done under medical supervision.

Some medications, like **benzodiazepines,** can cause serious withdrawal effects if stopped too abruptly. Muscle tension, dizziness, weakness, and a delightful little side dish of full-blown panic attacks can all result from an improperly managed taper (Vinkers et al., 2024).

So, while my experience suggests that suddenly removing a pile of medications might have been one of the catalysts for my turnaround, it's not a one-size-fits-all solution.

So, What Really Happened?

Despite the risks of sudden withdrawal, removing multiple medications may have given my brain the breathing room it desperately needed.

For years, my mind had been clouded, sedated, and trapped beneath the weight of polypharmacy. When hospice yanked those drugs away, it was as if a switch had been flipped. Slowly, my cognition began to clear.

But does this mean every person with dementia should stop taking all their medications?

Absolutely ***not***.

I'm not a doctor, and I certainly don't recommend haphazardly playing pharmacist.

What I do believe, though, is that in certain cases, medication overload might be making cognitive decline worse. If someone you love is on multiple prescriptions and their symptoms keep getting worse, deprescribing may be worth exploring—but only with the guidance of a competent, knowledgeable healthcare provider.

Because let's be honest: the last thing anyone needs is another medical crisis caused by a well-intentioned but misguided attempt at playing Dr. House.

2. The Starvation Factor

Losing over 100 pounds wasn't some well-planned, doctor-approved weight loss journey. There was no trendy meal plan, no motivational "before and after" photos—just a complete inability to eat, paired with the lingering certainty that all food had somehow turned to molten lava.

Looking back, I believe my extreme food aversion wasn't due to anorexia nervosa, where body image plays a role, but rather **Avoidant/Restrictive Food Intake Disorder (ARFID)**—a condition in which the brain irrationally rejects food due to sensory or psychological reasons. In my case, my mind had declared war on nourishment without any logic to back it up.

But here's where things get interesting. As miserable as my starvation was, it might have triggered a biological process that actually helped my brain heal.

Could Starvation Have Triggered a Brain Detox?

When the body isn't getting enough nutrients, it doesn't just shut down in defeat. It activates a built-in survival mechanism known as **autophagy**—a process where cells break down and recycle old, damaged components to stay functional. Essentially, it's the body's way of taking out the cellular trash.

Autophagy doesn't just impact muscle and organ tissue—it has been increasingly linked to brain health. Some studies suggest that this process may  help clear out diseased neurons and toxic protein clumps, which are known culprits in neurodegenerative diseases like Alzheimer's, Parkinson's, and Lewy body dementia (Guo et al., 2018).

And then there's **mitophagy,** a specialized version of autophagy that focuses on recycling malfunctioning **mitochondria** (the energy producers of our cells). When mitochondria become damaged, they produce **oxidative stress and neuronal inflammation**—a dangerous combination that accelerates brain deterioration. Research suggests that when mitophagy isn't working properly, these defective mitochondria accumulate, contributing to the progression of neurodegenerative diseases (Antico et al., 2025).

So, did my period of extreme starvation force my body to clear out diseased cells and reset my neurological function? It's a compelling theory—one that makes my reluctant hunger strike seem far more productive than I had ever imagined.

The Science Behind Starvation and Brain Repair

It sounds counterintuitive, but research has increasingly shown that periods of nutrient deprivation can trigger mechanisms that protect and enhance brain function. When cells are deprived of their usual supply of glucose and amino acids, they don't just wither away in despair. Instead, they enter survival mode, breaking down old, damaged components and recycling them for energy.

This process eliminates toxic proteins and defective neurons, potentially slowing or even reversing neurodegenerative damage (Fujikake et al., 2018).

Recent studies have shown that **intermittent fasting**—a controlled approach to scheduled eating—can improve cognitive function, enhance brain plasticity, and even help delay the onset of dementia by making brain cells more resilient and adaptable (Dong et al., 2024). While my own version of fasting was anything but controlled (or enjoyable), the underlying biological effects may have been the same.

So, Should You Starve Your Loved One with Dementia?

Absolutely *not*. Let's be very clear: extreme starvation is *dangerous*. Sudden, severe weight loss can lead to muscle wasting, organ damage, and a weakened immune system. It is not a recommended strategy for healing the brain.

However, there is growing evidence that controlled intermittent fasting, when done correctly and under proper medical supervision, may have cognitive benefits. Some researchers believe that periodic fasting may help reduce brain inflammation, clear toxic proteins, and enhance neural regeneration. But it's a delicate balance—one that should never be attempted without professional oversight.

A Body Smarter Than a Brain on Fire

Looking back, my unintentional experiment with starvation-induced autophagy might have been one of the factors that allowed my brain to hit the reset button. If my body was able to clear out cellular debris, eliminate harmful proteins, and kickstart neurological repair, then it wasn't just surviving—it was actively *fighting* for me.

The irony isn't lost on me. The very thing that nearly killed me might have also played a role in giving me back my mind.

While more research is needed to fully understand the link between fasting and cognitive function, my experience serves as a reminder that sometimes the body has its own way of healing, even when the mind isn't fully on board.

And in my case? My body might have just been smarter than I was all along.

3. My NDE: The Moment That Changed Everything

For months, I had been slipping further and further away. My body was shutting down, my mind was unraveling, and I was at the final stop. At that point, I wasn't questioning *if* I would die, but **when**. I had stopped eating, stopped moving—stopped existing in any meaningful way. For all intents and purposes, I was simply waiting for the inevitable.

But then, something extraordinary happened—something that flipped the entire script.

I had a **near-death experience (NDE)**—a moment so profound, so utterly real, that it changed *everything*. It wasn't a hallucination or a morphine-induced fever dream. I felt myself *leave my body*.

I didn't see the stereotypical "bright light" or hear the voices of lost loved ones. Instead, I was floating in an endless, deep blue sky, stars stretching out in every direction. It was peaceful, weightless, and unlike anything I had ever experienced before.

I truly believed I had transcended the material world and entered a realm of pure serenity.

In that moment, I wasn't sick. I wasn't weak. I wasn't struggling.

I simply *was*.

Then came the voice.

Not a booming command from the heavens, not a whisper from some unseen presence—but a thought, beamed directly into my mind. Strong, undeniable, almost magnetic in its force:

"It's not your time yet. You need to go back and help others with your experience."

It wasn't a suggestion. It was a directive.

And just like that, I knew—I had to fight my way back.

But here's where it gets interesting. This wasn't just a mental shift. My brain was physically changing during this experience, as if something inside me had been activated, reset, or rewired.

DMT: The Brain's Secret Survival Mechanism

Scientists believe that during an NDE, the brain floods itself with **N,N-Dimethyltryptamine (DMT)**—a powerful psychedelic compound naturally produced in small amounts but released in large doses during life-threatening situations, like when a person is dying.

DMT creates vivid, otherworldly experiences—often accompanied by profound peace, clarity, and euphoria. Some researchers even propose that DMT can stimulate **neuroplasticity,** the brain's ability to reorganize and form new neural pathways (*Near-Death Experiences*, 2021).

In other words, that surge of DMT during my NDE may have done more than just give me a beautiful vision—it might have *rebooted my brain.*

Think of it like a computer system crashing—stuck in a loop, overheating, unable to function. An NDE, with its flood of DMT and altered consciousness, may be the brain's last-ditch attempt to restart itself.

Was that what happened to me?

Terminal Lucidity: The Brain's Last Hurrah?

Another fascinating phenomenon that may have played a role in my turnaround is **terminal lucidity**—a sudden and often unexpected return of mental clarity in individuals with severe neurological conditions just before death.

Though the exact mechanisms remain a mystery, it suggests that the brain retains a hidden capacity for resilience, even in its final moments (Wikipedia contributors, 2025).

Some theories suggest that, as the body begins shutting down, a shift in brain chemistry or a **surge of neural activity** allows previously diminished cognitive abilities to resurface.

Whatever the cause, terminal lucidity challenges the assumption that neurodegenerative diseases completely erase a person's cognitive functions. Instead, it hints at the brain's untapped ability to restore lost functions—even when all logic says it shouldn't be possible.

Rewiring My Brain: The Will to Live Takes Over

As I returned to my body, something shifted.

My brain—once locked in a downward spiral, deteriorating with no apparent way out—suddenly seemed to *wake up.* It was as if it recognized there was still work to do, that it wasn't ready to shut down completely.

My will to live, buried for so long under layers of exhaustion, learned helplessness, and dementia-like fog, suddenly ignited—like a fire smoldering beneath the ashes.

This wasn't just about survival.

This was adaptation.

I believe this was neuroplasticity in action—the brain's extraordinary ability to reorganize, heal, and form new pathways when faced with trauma.

Science tells us that **neurodivergent brains**—those with autism, ADHD, or dyslexia—often develop alternative pathways to process and navigate challenges. Could my brain, in a desperate fight for survival, have tapped into similar mechanisms, rerouting itself to find a way forward?

Everything I thought I knew about cognitive decline told me that once the brain starts slipping, it only goes one way.

But that wasn't what happened.

I was supposed to be on an irreversible path to oblivion. Instead, my brain fought back. And that's the thing—*we don't fully understand what the brain is capable of.*

At first, the changes were subtle.

I wanted food again—something I hadn't cared about in ages. I started moving. Thinking. Reality, which had been slipping further and further away, became clearer.

The hallucinations—visions of shifting shadows, terrifying distortions of the world—began to fade. My speech improved. My memories, once lost in the abyss, started resurfacing.

But the biggest change?

I stood up.

Compassion as a Catalyst: The Moment I Chose to Stand

Not because I wanted to.

Not because I thought I could.

But because I felt sorry for my caregivers.

These kind, patient souls—some of them petite, struggling to lift me—were doing everything in their power to care for me. Tony, my CNA, was strong, but not everyone was built like him.

And one day, as I watched them strain to move me, I felt something I hadn't felt in a very long time—compassion for someone else's suffering.

That day, I didn't will myself to stand for me.

I did it for *them.*

Mind Over Matter: How Emotional Reintegration Played a Role

Beyond the chemical and neurological changes, there was another crucial factor: **Connection**.

One of the most overlooked aspects of dementia and end-of-life care is the devastating impact of isolation. When we are cut off from the world—physically, emotionally, mentally—it accelerates cognitive decline.

Once I started engaging again—once I had a purpose, a reason to keep going—my brain began to *thrive*.

It's no secret that social interaction stimulates cognitive function, but for me, reconnecting with the world wasn't just beneficial—it was *essential*.

The emotional reintegration, the sense of purpose that had once seemed so far out of reach, became just as vital as the physical changes happening in my brain.

My will to keep going wasn't just about survival anymore.

It wasn't just about proving that I could defy the odds.

It was about the people I could help, the knowledge I could pass on, and the story that, against all logic, I was still here to tell.

From Actively Dying to Actively Living

If you had asked anyone—including myself—whether I would survive those final days in hospice, the answer would have been an emphatic **"No."**

I was too far gone, too sick, too lost in the fog of neurodegeneration.

But something inside me—whether it was the NDE, the DMT release, neuroplasticity, or sheer willpower—refused to let me go.

My brain rewired itself.

My body, once frail and starved, began to strengthen.

My mind, once consumed by confusion, started to clear.

Science doesn't fully understand why some people experience near-miraculous turnarounds while others don't.

But I do know this: I was given a *choice*.

And I chose to live.

4. Releasing the Weight of Trauma

For decades, I carried my trauma like an invisible weight pressing down on me—so deeply embedded that I barely recognized it was there. It wasn't just mental; it was physical, too. Trauma has a way of entrenching itself in the body, shaping how we move, how we react, and even how we experience pain.

Dr. Bessel van der Kolk, one of the leading researchers on trauma and author of _The Body Keeps the Score_, explains that trauma isn't just a memory—it's stored in the nervous system, muscles, and even our immune response. It imprints itself onto the body, subtly shifting the way we breathe, stand, sleep, and even digest food. Trauma doesn't just haunt the past—it lives in the present.

For years, I had been living in a body hijacked by a lifetime of distress, grief, and unresolved emotional pain. But when I was placed in hospice, and all of my curative medications were abruptly stopped, something _changed_. It was as if my body finally had a chance to process the very things it had been suppressing for so long.

My brain, no longer sedated or numbed, had to confront what had been lingering beneath the surface. The combination of medication withdrawal, my near-death experience, and my sheer will to survive may have given my body the opening it needed to reset.

The Science Behind Trauma and the Body

Dr. van der Kolk describes trauma as something that "lives in the body." It isn't just a memory we replay in our minds; it's a physiological experience that lingers long after the traumatic event has passed.

Trauma _rewires_ the brain, particularly in areas like the **amygdala** (the fear center of the brain) and the **prefrontal cortex** (which helps regulate emotions and decision-making). Over time, a traumatized brain stays in a hyper-alert state, constantly expecting danger, even when none is present.

This is why many people who experience trauma suffer from chronic stress, anxiety, and even physical pain for years—not because the event is still happening, but because the body _never got the signal that it was over._

Dr. van der Kolk's groundbreaking research challenges the conventional view that trauma is purely psychological. Instead, he reveals that trauma is deeply embedded in both the mind and body, shaping everything from emotional responses to physical health. His work emphasizes that unresolved trauma doesn't just linger in memories—it _imprints itself_ on the nervous system, muscles, and even organ function, often manifesting as chronic pain, immune dysfunction, and other health issues (*The Body Keeps the Score*, n.d.).

One of van der Kolk's most powerful assertions is that traditional talk therapy and medications often fall short in fully addressing trauma's impact. While they may help manage symptoms, they don't resolve the physiological scars that trauma leaves behind.

He famously stated, "*Pills don't heal trauma,*" underscoring the limitations of medication in treating deeply rooted emotional wounds. Instead, he advocates for body-based therapies—such as movement, breathwork, and sensory experiences—that allow the body to release stored trauma and reestablish a sense of safety (Luscombe, 2024).

In my case, the abrupt cessation of medications in hospice might have created the space for my body to engage in its natural healing processes. Without the constant interference of pharmaceuticals, my system had the freedom to process and release the deep-seated trauma it had been holding onto for years.

Through somatic healing, I became more attuned to my body's signals, gradually fostering a sense of safety within myself that had long been absent. This process allowed me to confront and integrate old wounds, not just mentally but physically.

Perhaps, by finally addressing the toll of past trauma, my body was able to regain its strength and function in ways no one thought possible.

Somatic Healing and Trauma Release

Somatic healing focuses on reconnecting the mind and body. Instead of just talking about trauma, it involves physical practices that help process emotions trapped inside the body.

Some common somatic therapies include:

- **Breathwork** – Deep, intentional breathing helps calm the nervous system and release stored tension.
- **Movement Therapy** – Activities like yoga or even simple stretching can help the body process trauma.
- **Touch Therapy** – Gentle physical touch (like massage or certain therapeutic techniques) can help regulate the nervous system.

- **Vocal Expression** – Making sounds, humming, or singing can stimulate the **vagus nerve** (the longest cranial nerve, connecting various organs along the path from your brainstem down to your digestive system), which plays a key role in regulating stress and trauma responses.

Even though I wasn't consciously engaging in these therapies while in hospice, my body may have been instinctively doing some of them on its own.

Perhaps the weight loss I experienced triggered my nervous system to enter a state of "self-preservation," where it was forced to repair itself at a cellular level.

Maybe my near-death experience, where I felt an overwhelming sense of peace, acted as a reset for my trauma-riddled brain.

Was This the Missing Piece in My Healing?

Looking back, I wonder if I had been trapped in a cycle where my trauma, medications, and declining health were feeding into each other. Each layer added more dysfunction to my body, making true healing nearly impossible.

But when all of that was stripped away—the medications, the constant fear of dying, and even my attachment to my old self—my body finally had the space to heal.

Dr. van der Kolk's work suggests that people who process trauma through the body often experience profound healing, even when traditional therapies have failed.

So, is it possible that my mind and body, when given the right circumstances, did what it had been trying to do all along?

Could my transformation have been my body's last-ditch effort to survive, to heal, and to rewrite the ending of my story?

One thing is undeniable—what happened to me isn't supposed to happen.

My turnaround defies traditional medical expectations, yet when viewed through the lens of trauma, neuroscience, and somatic healing, the pieces start to fit.

CHAPTER 26: EXPLAINING THE UNEXPLAINABLE

So, let's dig deep here and finalize these theories. How, exactly, do you explain the unexplainable?

One day, I was actively dying. Not in the poetic sense—not in the way people say they feel "dead inside" during grief or heartbreak—but in the stark, medical, hospice-confirmed sense of the word. I had stopped eating. Stopped speaking. Stopped moving. My body was shutting down, my mind unraveling, and my family had already made arrangements for my cremation. The world had counted me out.

And yet, here I am. Fully. Completely. Unmistakably alive.

Not just functioning. Not just surviving. *Living.*

My cognition returned. My strength returned. My sense of self—something I had lost so completely I never thought I'd find it again—came crashing back with such force that even my doctors are still trying to make sense of it.

The truth is, modern medicine has no category for people like me. There is no checkbox for "terminally ill patient defies prognosis and regains full cognitive and motor function." According to the textbooks, people with advanced neurodegeneration don't just *wake up* one day and start thinking, speaking, and walking again.

And yet, that's exactly what I did.

What Was My Actual Diagnosis?

That's the mystery, isn't it?

My probable diagnosis was Lewy body dementia (LBD), and I matched nearly every symptom. I had 30 out of 34 clinical markers—hallucinations, tremors, autonomic dysfunction, Capgras syndrome, delusions. And yet, LBD is a progressive, irreversible disease. No one wakes up one day and simply *doesn't* have it anymore.

Frontotemporal dementia (FTD) had also been considered years earlier. That diagnosis still terrifies me. FTD doesn't just take memory—it dismantles personality, impulse control, and human connection. It turns you into someone unrecognizable, someone unable to feel empathy, to regulate behavior, to interact with the world in any meaningful way. If I had FTD, and somehow my brain *reversed* it, then my case should be front-page medical news.

Could it have been drug-induced Parkinsonism from years of psychiatric medications? Maybe. But that doesn't explain the years of decline *before* I was ever put on those drugs.

Could it have been pseudodementia—severe depression mimicking cognitive decline? Possibly. But my symptoms weren't just psychological; they were profoundly, unmistakably *physical*.

Was it a rare, undiagnosed neurological syndrome? A combination of multiple conditions compounded by medication, trauma, and sheer neurological misfortune?

The truth is, I may never have a definitive answer. And maybe that's okay.

Because sometimes, when science can't explain something, it simply means **we haven't caught up to the truth yet**.

The Science is Catching Up

We're starting to learn that the brain is far more resilient than we ever imagined. Concepts like neuroplasticity—the brain's ability to rewire itself—are proving to be powerful forces in cognitive health. Autophagy and mitophagy—the body's mechanisms for clearing out damaged cells and regenerating healthy ones—are becoming recognized as key players in longevity and disease reversal.

And then there are the emerging breakthroughs. Scientists at the University of Southampton recently developed a laser-based test that can detect early signs of dementia with just a drop of bodily fluid—years before symptoms even

appear (Shaw, 2024). Imagine what that could mean. Earlier intervention. More effective treatments. A future where people don't just decline into dementia but have a fighting chance to stop it before it starts.

So, what if my *impossible* turnaround isn't just some anomaly? What if it holds the key to something we don't fully understand yet? What if my case challenges the belief that neurodegeneration is always a one-way street?

Maybe it Really *Was* All in My Head

There's a phrase that's been tossed around throughout my transformative journey—one that, for most people, is laced with condescension, invalidation, and frustration.

"Maybe it's all in your head."

I heard it from doctors. From people who didn't believe my symptoms. From those who thought I was exaggerating, making it up, or simply being difficult. And for a long time, I hated that phrase.

But now?

Now I realize... maybe they were **right**.

Just not in the way they thought.

Because, what if *it really was **all in my head***—not in the sense that it was imaginary, but in the sense that my brain *was* the battleground all along? What if the key to my so-called *impossible* comeback wasn't outside of me but **within** me?

What if my brain, when given the right circumstances—whether through neuroplasticity, autophagy, somatic healing, or sheer willpower—*rewired itself* to fight its way back?

Because the mind is powerful. The brain can adapt, change, and find new pathways. And sometimes, when the medical world says, *"There's nothing more we can do,"* the brain responds, *"Oh, yeah? **Watch me**."*

A Perfect Storm—or a Miracle?

If you're looking for a single explanation for my return from the brink, I can't give you one. Because it wasn't just *one* thing. It was everything.

- The abrupt removal of psychiatric and neurological medications, which may have allowed my brain to reset itself.

- A prolonged period of starvation that could have triggered deep cellular detox and repair.

- A near-death experience that may have flooded my brain with DMT, a naturally occurring psychedelic linked to neuroplasticity and cognitive breakthroughs.

- Somatic healing, allowing my body to finally process and release decades of stored trauma.

- The power of human connection—my compassion for the caregivers who refused to abandon me, the family members who fought for me, and my sheer determination to get better so I could help *others*.

And then there's the last possibility—the one some people might scoff at, but I can't ignore.

Maybe, just maybe, it was a **miracle**.

Because let's be honest: I *shouldn't* be here. But I am.

And if that doesn't shake the foundations of what we think we know about life, death, and the human spirit—what will?

Miracles, Mistakes, and Masterpieces

Now, listen closely—there's one more thing I need you to understand.

I have made more mistakes in my life than I can count. Some small. Some catastrophic. The kind of mistakes that should have been the *end* of me.

But if there's one surprising lesson I've learned throughout my 88 years around the sun, it's this:

Miracles don't belong to the perfect.

They don't wait for the saintly, the deserving, the ones who have it all figured out. They find the broken. The lost. The ones who have fallen so far they can't see a way back. And somehow, against all odds, they rise.

And here's the real truth about miracles:

They don't just happen *to* us. They happen *through* us.

Through the caregivers who show up, exhausted but determined. Through the family members who keep fighting battles no one else sees. Through the kindness of strangers who choose compassion when no one is watching.

And through **you**.

Do you know what it took to make you? Every cell in your body carries the imprint of generations before you. Every strand of your DNA is an unbroken thread tying you to those who came before—those who fought, those who endured, those who refused to let the story end.

So, if you take nothing else from this book, take this:

No matter how lost you feel, no matter how many times you stumble, you are not beyond hope.

You are not beyond redemption.

You are a **masterpiece**, not a disasterpiece.

And don't you ever forget it.

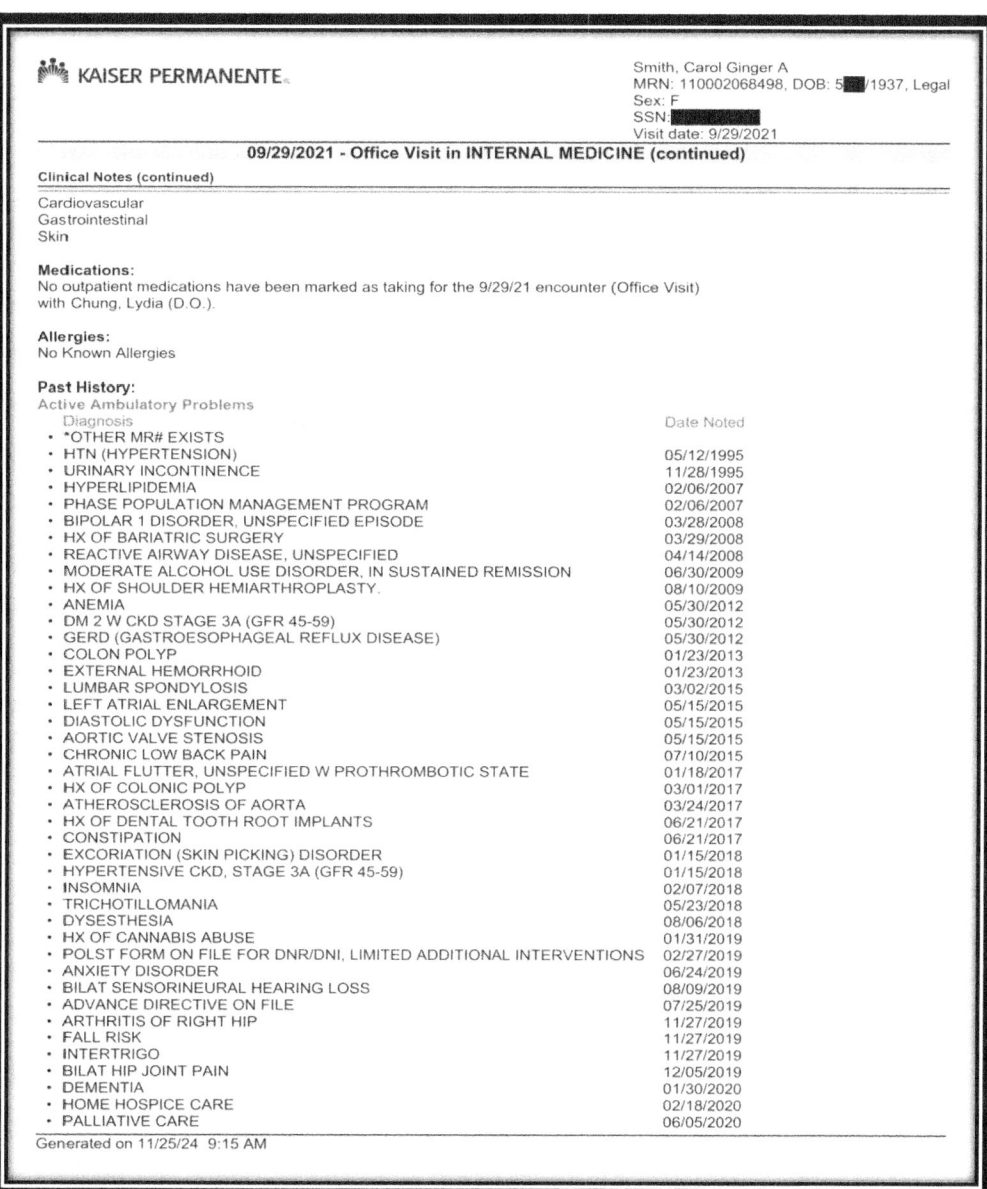

List of Medical Diagnoses History

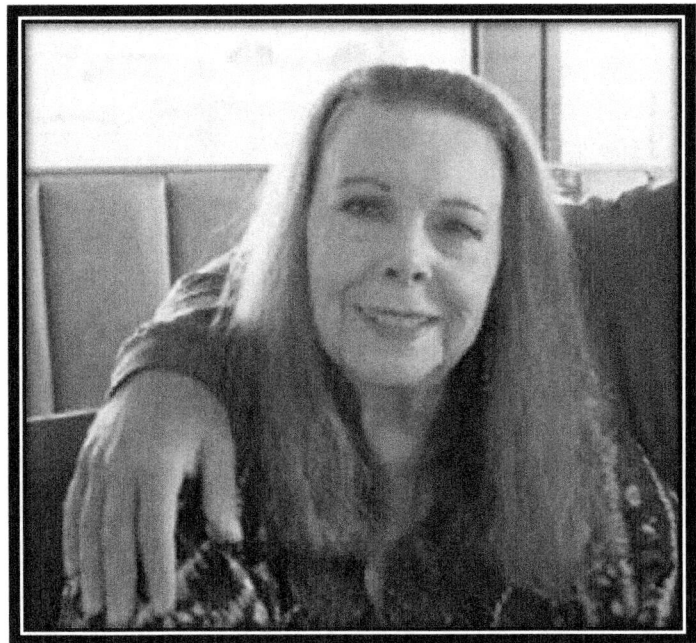

Me, before hospice

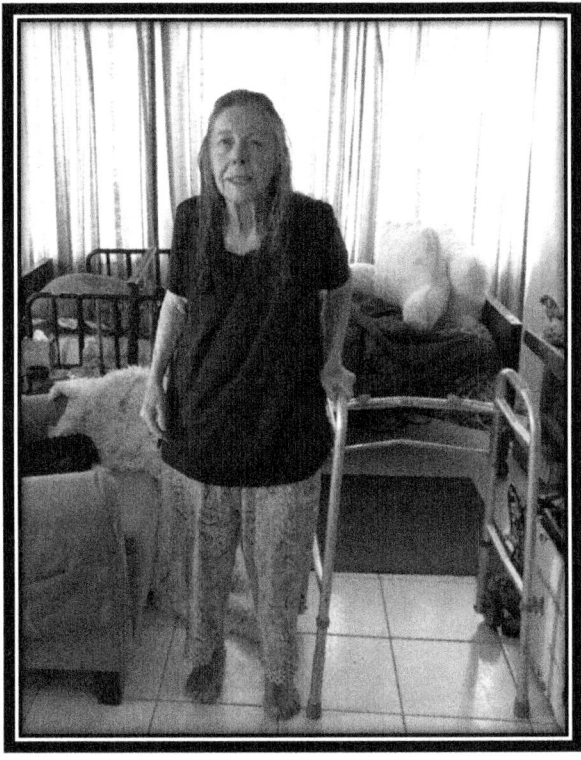

Me, after hospice

CONCLUSION: YOUR STORY ISN'T OVER YET

In 2018, I was handed what amounted to an eviction notice from life—seven years, they told me. Seven years to fade, seven years before dementia swallowed me whole. Doctors spoke as if my fate was already sealed, a slow, merciless countdown to nothingness.

But somehow, I lived past my expiration date.

Not by accident. Not by luck. And not even by sheer will alone.

Somewhere in the abyss, when I should have been slipping away, something happened. A near-death experience. A moment so vivid and undeniable that it changed everything. Maybe it was divine intervention. Maybe it was a one-in-a-billion neurological fluke. Maybe it was just sheer stubbornness refusing to go quietly.

Whatever it was, it pulled me back and set me on a path I never could have imagined.

And so, I fought.

I clawed my way out of the darkness—through trauma, through suffering, through all the mistakes and regrets that should have buried me. Every rational reason said I shouldn't be here. But I am. And not just alive—I'm thriving.

Teepa Snow, one of the world's leading dementia experts, once called me a "unicorn" in one of our interviews. She also said something else that has never left me:

"Not many people would choose to come back from the brink of death the way you did. It would have been so much easier to just let go."

And she's right. It *would* have been easier. But I didn't let go.

Because something—or someone—told me there was a story that needed to be told.

But this isn't just my story.

This is a message.

A message for those who have been dismissed, abandoned, or written off. A message for anyone who has ever been told they are too broken, too lost, too far gone.

I am here to tell you—***you are not beyond saving***. You are not beyond hope.

I have survived horrors that should have destroyed me—addiction, misdiagnosis, overmedication, systemic failure, and the slow, merciless descent into dementia. I walked right up to the edge of death, felt its quiet pull, and then—against all odds—turned back.

And what I learned, what I lived, is that maybe it really was *all in my head*—just not in the way the doctors thought.

When they said it dismissively, they meant I was imagining my symptoms, that I was exaggerating, that my suffering wasn't real. But the truth is, my healing **was** in my head—not as a delusion, but as a biological reality. My brain was capable of rewiring itself, of adapting, of finding a way through the darkness when all seemed lost.

So, if you've ever been told that your pain, your illness, or your struggle is "all in your head," I urge you to reframe it. Maybe the answer really is inside of you—not as something to dismiss, but as something to explore.

Your brain is not static. Your body is not beyond change. The human mind and body hold untapped potential for healing that even modern medicine cannot fully explain.

The Path to Healing: How You Can Start Your Own Journey

I don't claim to have all the answers. But what I do know is that the way we approach healing needs to change. The body and brain are not separate entities; they work together. And if my experience has taught me anything, it's that true healing is never just *one* thing.

Take care of yourself. Nourish your mind. Move, breathe, connect with others, and give your brain every possible advantage. Because I truly believe that one day, there *will be a cure* for dementia. Maybe not in my lifetime, but perhaps in yours. And when that cure arrives, you'll want to be in the best shape possible—ready to embrace it, ready to thrive.

If you're reading this and wondering, *"Where do I even begin?"*—let me tell you: **Start with your body**.

1. Ground Yourself in the Present. Your nervous system needs safety before it can heal. Simple grounding techniques—pressing your feet onto the floor, touching something cold, or focusing on your breath—can signal to your body that it is safe, allowing it to shift out of survival mode (Aybar, 2021).

2. Reconnect with Your Body Through Movement. Whether it's stretching, walking, or even just swaying to music, movement tells your brain that you are alive, engaged, and capable of change. Gentle movement-based therapies like tai chi, yoga, or dance can help integrate trauma stored in the body and improve neural connections (Barhum, 2024).

3. Harness the Power of Your Breath. Deep, intentional breathing can calm the nervous system and regulate emotions. Techniques like diaphragmatic breathing or humming (which stimulates the vagus nerve) can help your body move out of a stress response and into a state of repair.

4. Engage in Somatic Healing. Trauma and illness leave imprints on the body. Somatic therapies—such as body scans, trauma-release exercises, and gentle massage—can help process emotions trapped within the body (*Somatic Self Care*, n.d.).

5. Reduce External Stressors. Chronic stress fuels neurodegeneration. Mindfulness, meditation, and spending time in nature have been shown to decrease inflammation in the brain and promote cognitive resilience (Blumberg, 2024).

6. Reevaluate Medications with Your Doctor. While medications can be lifesaving, unnecessary or excessive prescriptions can also contribute to cognitive decline. If you suspect that your medications may be affecting your brain function, talk to a trusted doctor or pharmacist about deprescribing options. (I go into this in more detail in Bonus #1: My Personal Tips for Caregivers, which you can download from this **LINK**.)

7. Nourish Your Brain. Food plays a massive role in brain health. Reducing processed foods, increasing healthy fats (like omega-3s), and prioritizing anti-inflammatory nutrients can support cognitive function and longevity.

8. Seek Connection. Isolation is one of the biggest contributors to cognitive decline. Find ways to stay engaged—through support groups, volunteering, or simply reaching out to a friend. Even small acts of social engagement can keep the brain active and resilient.

9. Challenge the Idea That Decline is Inevitable. Science is catching up to what many of us already feel in our bones: The brain can change. Neuroplasticity is real. Healing *is possible*.

And if I can stand here today telling you this after being written off as terminal—***then maybe it's possible for you, too.***

EPILOGUE

From Barking Like a Dog to Finding My Voice

Today, I am thrilled to say I am leading a fulfilled life—one rich in purpose and connections. Through my advocacy, I've found a sense of community and belonging. I've had the opportunity to participate in dementia training programs, engage in public speaking, give countless interviews, serve on boards of numerous activist initiatives, and contribute to meaningful causes.

When I'm not advocating, exposing scammers, or participating in clinical trials (which some would call "prostituting my body for science," but I call "earning my keep"), you'll find me enjoying self-care with creative arts, exploring new crafts, or taking in the beauty of nature around my beloved lagoon.

I am profoundly grateful for the love and support of my family members who have reconnected with me, as well as the kindness of volunteers who have helped me along the way. I want to give a shout-out to the helpers of my blog and social media platforms—without them, I'd probably still be locked out of my own accounts.

I am also thankful that I am able to share my story, raise awareness, and connect with others who are passionate about creating a better world. For professionals, caregivers, and support workers, I urge you to approach your work with empathy and understanding. See the humanity in the people you support, the intricate web of relationships surrounding them, and the dignity they still possess, even when dementia tries to strip it away.

I am committed to shedding light on the imperfections within the medical system and to breaking down stigmas through understanding and empowerment.

From barking like a dog in the depths of dementia's darkness to living a life filled with purpose, my journey—once marked by the threads of dementia, trauma, and addiction—has now given rise to a powerful voice—poignant for me as a former speech-language pathologist.

Whether my turnaround was due to a physical transformation, a near-death experience, or something beyond explanation, I may never know. But what I do know is this—reclaiming my life from dementia defied every expectation. Sharing my story matters because if it happened to me, who's to say it couldn't happen to someone else? If my journey proves anything, it's that healing is possible, even when the world has already written you off.

Getting My Message Out

At 88, I don't have time to waste. There's still work to be done, still battles to fight, still stories to tell. My unique life purpose has become my platform, my odyssey of healing and resilience a bridge to help others. I share what I've learned—not out of self-indulgence, but to raise awareness, ignite conversation, and (hopefully) ensure that no one else has to endure what I did without hope.

If you'd like to stay in touch or take a peek at more highlights of my journey, you can email me at: Gingerspeech@gmail.com or find me on Instagram at: @gingersmith104

I'm also excited about participating in various podcast interviews about my experience. Here are some of the ones I've done in the past, but keep your eyes open for more of these once this book is published:

Teepa Snow / Website: https://teepasnow.com

Teepa's site offers exceptional video lectures on YouTube, books, and classes on dementia care. You can find my two interviews (so far) with Teepa Snow on YouTube.

The first one premiered in September of 2022 and can be found at this link: https://www.youtube.com/watch?v=4vrY5RRQvuo

The second one premiered in April of 2024 and can be found at this link:

https://www.youtube.com/watch?v=Izm_TAQbjwc

Positive Aging Community / Website:

https://retirementlivingsourcebook.com

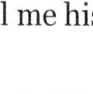

Founded by Steve Gurney in 1990, this site connects older adults, families, and professionals with essential resources for aging well. It also provides comprehensive listings of retirement housing, aging-in-place options, and supportive services. Steve has interviewed me twice since I returned home from the board and care facility, and he continues to call me his "favorite guest" on his YouTube channel.

Our first interview took place in May of 2023, and you can find it at this link: https://www.youtube.com/watch?v=AjipANNdHBQ

And then, in March of 2024, I joined Steve for another update on my post-dementia journey. You can find that interview at this link:

https://www.youtube.com/watch?v=r8A84bfzYLI

Alzheimer's Speaks / Website:

https://alzheimersspeaks.com/

An advocacy organization founded by Lori La Bey (named as a "Health Hero" by Oprah Winfrey), dedicated to shifting dementia care from crisis to comfort through education, support, and global collaboration. Offering resources like  the Alzheimer's Speaks Radio podcast, Dementia Chats™ videos, and the Dementia Map resource directory, it connects caregivers, professionals, and those living with dementia to valuable tools and community support.

Watch my interview with Lori from January 2024 at this link:

https://www.youtube.com/watch?v=az3aErT2tKA

The Dementia Action Alliance has posted a short video on their website titled "Tips for Communication and Connection," in which I am interviewed. You can watch it here:

https://www.youtube.com/watch?v=vgK7VofdO1M

I was also honored to be featured in this four-minute video about loneliness on the Peninsula Family Service website: https://vimeo.com/911333235

Plus, in May of 2024, I had the pleasure of participating in an interview with Einav Avni on her *Healing Conversations* YouTube channel. You can find that here: https://www.youtube.com/watch?v=6iHlRbXwrEk

I've also started a blog about my journey, and I will do my best to update it from time to time. It's been a work in progress that I hope to master very soon. If you'd like to take a peek, here's the link:

https://gingerspeech.wixsite.com/my-site-1

But don't think for a second that I'm slowing down—there's still so much work to be done. The number of people affected by dementia is growing faster than ever, and too many are left without a voice, without support, and without hope.

So, if you're willing, I invite you to stand with me—to advocate, to educate, and to fight for those who can no longer fight for themselves. Because I truly believe that together, we **can and will** make a difference.

BONUS #1: My Personal Tips for Caregivers

Caregiving isn't just a job or a duty—it's a full-blown, life-altering experience that demands everything you have and then asks for more. I know this because I've lived it from every possible angle.

As a retired speech-language pathologist, former rehab manager, trained nursing attendant, hands-on care aide, and caregiver myself, I've been in the trenches—witnessing firsthand the heartbreak, the exhaustion, and the overwhelming weight of responsibility that comes with caring for someone with dementia.

But I've also seen the resilience, the unexpected moments of joy, and the deep, unshakable bonds that make it all worthwhile.

Whether you're a family caregiver trying to balance it all, a home care provider giving everything you've got, or a professional in the field, I want to offer you something more than just survival tactics. I want to share real, practical insights—the kind that come from both sides of the caregiving equation.

Because here's the truth: caring for someone with dementia is unpredictable, often unfair, and undeniably exhausting. But with the right tools, strategies, and mindset, it can also be a path of growth, strength, and even moments of profound connection.

So, let's get into it. What follows isn't theory—it's the real deal. Hard-earned lessons, workarounds, and personal tips from someone who's been there, done that, and, against all odds, lived to tell the tale.

My hope is that these insights will lighten your load, strengthen your resolve, and, most importantly, remind you that your well-being *matters* too.

Download this 30+ page list of my own personalized tips for caregivers from this LINK.

BONUS #2: My Advice to Help You Navigate the Healthcare System and Avoid Scammers & Charlatans

Here's something I've come to realize: surviving dementia is only half the battle. The other half? Navigating a healthcare system that often seems rigged against us, dodging scammers and charlatans, and fighting tooth and nail to get the care we actually need. I've been through it all—the denials, the runarounds, the endless bureaucratic nonsense—and if there's one thing I want you to take away from my experience, it's that you have to be your own advocate. No one is going to fight harder for your well-being than you or your authorized caregiver.

Lately, public outrage over the state of our healthcare system has reached a boiling point, and for good reason. The shocking murder of UnitedHealthcare CEO Brian Thompson in December 2024 sent shockwaves through the industry and intensified scrutiny over insurance practices—particularly claim denials. Thompson's death, reportedly linked to an assailant who carried a manifesto criticizing the healthcare system, has reignited discussions about the growing frustration Americans feel toward insurance companies and the way they routinely deny coverage for necessary treatments.

And the numbers don't lie. In 2023 alone, insurers offering plans through HealthCare.gov denied 19% of in-network claims and a staggering 37% of out-of-network claims. Some plans rejected **_over half_** of all in-network claims (Lo et al., 2025). These aren't just statistics—they represent real people being denied essential care, forced to fight for the treatments their doctors have prescribed, or left drowning in medical debt.

The rise of automation in processing claims has only made things worse. AI-driven algorithms, designed to cut costs, are making snap decisions about who gets approved and who doesn't—often with little to no human oversight. What was once a frustrating but manageable process has become an uphill battle, discouraging people from even attempting to appeal.

This frustration isn't just theoretical; it's personal. I know what it feels like to be at the mercy of a system that doesn't seem to care whether you live or die. I spent years in facilities where the standard of care varied wildly. I've had treatments denied, essential medications stripped away, and decisions about my health made by people who never even met me.

I often wonder—was my survival a fluke, or is there something to learn from it? And if so, could that knowledge help others? These questions drive me, even as time works against me. At 88, with heart and kidney issues and a 50% chance of developing dementia again, I know that every day matters. I've lost so much—my mother, my daughter, my sense of self during my worst years—but I've also gained resilience, perspective, and a strength I never knew I had. I fought my way to sobriety. I learned to let go of fear and emotional chaos. And while the possibility of decline still lingers in the back of my mind, I choose gratitude instead of fear. I am here. I am still fighting.

But I also know that no one gets through this system unscathed unless they learn how to fight back. So, here's a taste of my advice—hard-earned wisdom from someone who's been chewed up and spat out by this industry more times than I can count:

- **Know your policy.** Read the fine print. Understand what your insurance covers and, more importantly, what it doesn't. Don't wait until you're in crisis mode to find out.

- **Keep records.** Every bill, every conversation, every denial letter—document everything. When they try to tell you something wasn't approved, you'll have the proof.

- **Challenge denials.** Don't assume that "no" is the final answer. Appeal and, if necessary, escalate your case. Insurance companies count on people giving up.

- **Ask questions.** If a doctor says something doesn't make sense or an insurer refuses a treatment, demand an explanation. You have a right to know why decisions are being made about your care.

- **Seek outside help.** If you hit a wall, contact your state's insurance commissioner or a patient advocacy group. You don't have to take on this fight alone.

More than 20 pages of healthcare insights and personal advice can be downloaded from this LINK, where I explain more about how to deal with the healthcare system, avoid scams, and advocate for yourself or your loved one. I hope it helps you find the clarity, confidence, and strength you need in a system that too often leaves people feeling lost.

Because in a world where medical decisions are increasingly dictated by profits and algorithms, we have to fight harder than ever to make sure we—and the people we love—get the care we deserve.

ALSO BY THE AUTHOR

In 2024, I published three books that were designed to complement each other in every step of dementia caregiving. I'd be honored if you would take a look at them because I truly believe they will be helpful in your caregiving duties.

"Dealing with Dementia for Caregivers" is your go-to guide (getting very high praise from caregivers) for real-world advice to manage daily challenges and provide the best care possible.

https://mybook.to/DEALINGWITHDEMENTIA

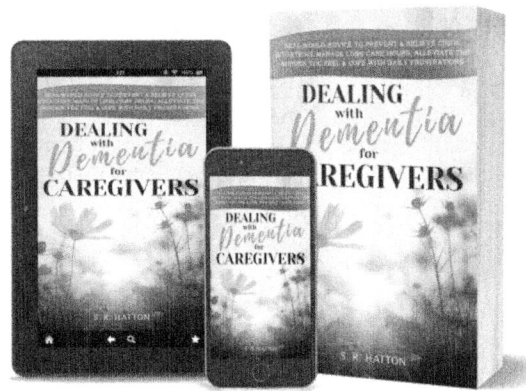

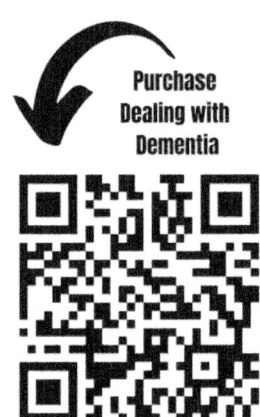

Purchase Dealing with Dementia

"Tales from Memory Lane" is a collection of large print short stories designed to entertain and engage seniors in reminiscence therapy.
https://mybook.to/TalesfromMemoryLane

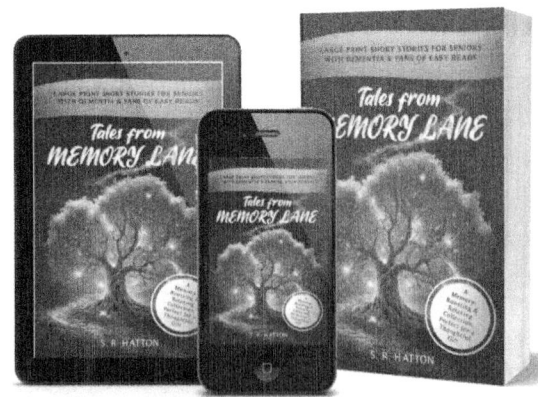

Purchase Tales from Memory Lane

"The Memory Keeper" is the ultimate memory-saving and medical detail-documenting guide, making it a sentimental (and practical) treasure for generations.

https://mybook.to/THEMEMORYKEEPER

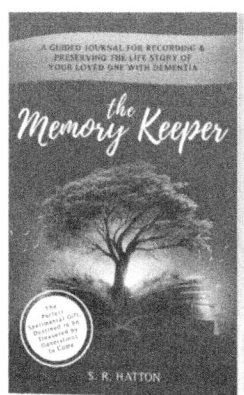

Together, these books offer comprehensive support and a heartfelt gesture for anyone navigating the tough journey of dementia caregiving. They're more than just books; they're tools of love meant to bring comfort and help during those challenging times.

ONE LAST REQUEST

"No one is useless in this world who lightens the burdens of another." — Charles Dickens

You've just traveled through the astonishing pages of *Dementia Denied: One Woman's True Story of Surviving a Terminal Diagnosis & Reclaiming Her Life*. Whether you laughed, cried, or found yourself nodding through the wild and winding chapters—you're now holding something powerful: perspective.

And what better way to give back than by paying it forward?

Your review could be the miracle someone else needs.

Every word you share—about the chapters that hit hardest, the moments that brought hope, or the tools you now carry—is a seed planted in the fertile soil of someone else's healing journey.

A new caregiver, a struggling patient, a weary family member... someone out there is searching for reassurance that *this isn't the end of their story either.*

Let's show them it's possible to rewrite fate.

Why Your Review Matters:

- **Leave a Legacy**
  - Just like Ginger, you've been changed by the story. Now you can help change someone else's. Your review becomes a ripple in a growing wave of hope.
- **Be the Light in the Fog**
  - Let others know which insights, humor, or hard truths helped you the most. Your words could be the flashlight in their darkest hour.
- **Grow the Garden of Shared Wisdom**
  - Each review contributes to a community of readers who are done being dismissed, gaslit, or overlooked—and who now know, without a doubt, that healing doesn't have to follow the rules.

Ready to Share Your Chapter?

Please, if you could spare just one more minute of your time, scan the QR code below to leave your review on Amazon. Whether it's a few heartfelt lines or a full reflection, your voice really does matter.

One last thing...

The author truly believes that one day there *will* be a cure for dementia. Maybe not in her lifetime—but maybe in yours. So, let's keep building bridges, not just for ourselves but for the generations to come. Start by lifting your voice.

Thank you for being part of this story.

Now, please help someone else start theirs.

Review
Dementia Denied

CITATION RESOURCES

10 Things You Should Know about LBD – Lewy Body Dementia Association. (n.d.). https://www.lbda.org/10-things-you-should-know-about-lbd

Antico, O., Thompson, P.W., Hertz, N.T. *et al. Targeting mitophagy in neurodegenerative diseases.* Nature Reviews Drug Discovery (2025). https://doi.org/10.1038/s41573-024-01105-0

Aybar, S. (2021, July 21). *4 Somatic Therapy Exercises for Healing from Trauma.* Psych Central. https://psychcentral.com/lib/somatic-therapy-exercises-for-trauma#grounding

Barhum, L. (2024, December 9). *7 easy somatic exercises for a healthier mind and body.* Verywell Health. https://www.verywellhealth.com/somatic-exercises-8749929

Blumberg, P. O. (2024, September 8). *Stressed? Here's how to engage your five senses to beat work worries.* New York Post. https://nypost.com/2024/09/08/lifestyle/stressed-heres-how-to-engage-your-five-senses-to-beat-work-worries/

Chippa, V., & Roy, K. (2023). *Geriatric Cognitive Decline and Polypharmacy.* In www.ncbi.nlm.nih.gov (No. NBK574575). StatPearls Publishing LLC. Retrieved February 2, 2025, from https://www.ncbi.nlm.nih.gov/books/NBK574575

Dong, H., Wang, S., Hu, C., Wang, M., Zhou, T., & Zhou, Y. (2024). *Neuroprotective effects of intermittent fasting in the aging brain.* Annals of Nutrition and Metabolism, 80(4), 175–185. https://doi.org/10.1159/000538782

Engel, B. (2024, September 17). *The Lesser-Known Effects of Childhood Sexual Abuse.* Psychology Today. https://www.psychologytoday.com/us/blog/the-compassion-chronicles/202409/the-lesser-known-effects-of-childhood-sexual-abuse

FastStats. (n.d.). Hospice Care. https://www.cdc.gov/nchs/fastats/hospice-care.htm

Fujikake, N., Shin, M., & Shimizu, S. (2018). *Association between autophagy and neurodegenerative diseases.* Frontiers in Neuroscience, 12. https://doi.org/10.3389/fnins.2018.00255

Guo, F., Liu, X., Cai, H., & Le, W. (2018). *Autophagy in neurodegenerative diseases: pathogenesis and therapy.* Brain pathology (Zurich, Switzerland), 28(1), 3–13. https://doi.org/10.1111/bpa.12545

INBrief: Early Childhood Mental health. (2020, October 29). Center on the Developing Child at Harvard University. https://developingchild.harvard.edu/resources/inbrief-early-childhood-mental-health/

Is there a shortage of speech-language pathologists? (n.d.). Zippia. https://www.zippia.com/answers/is-there-a-shortage-of-speech-language-pathologists/

Jeglic, E. L., PhD. (2021, May 6). *Psychological, physical, social and economic impacts of childhood sexual abuse.* Psychology Today. https://www.psychologytoday.com/us/blog/protecting-children-from-sexual-abuse/202105/the-long-lasting-consequences-of-child-sexual

LaChappelle, B. (2024, April 20). *5 Facts about lewy body dementia for family caregivers.* Integra Health. https://www.integrahomehealth.com/5-facts-about-lewy-body-dementia-for-family-caregivers

Lanzi, A. M., Ellison, J. M., & Cohen, M. L. (2021). *The "Counseling+" Roles of the Speech-Language Pathologist Serving Older Adults With Mild Cognitive Impairment and Dementia From Alzheimer's Disease.* Perspectives of the ASHA Special Interest Groups, 6(5), 987–1002. https://doi.org/10.1044/2021_persp-20-00295

Lo, J., Long, M., Wallace, R., Salaga, M., & Pestaina, K. (2025, February 3). *Claims denials and appeals in ACA Marketplace Plans in 2023 | KFF.* KFF. https://www.kff.org/private-insurance/issue-brief/claims-denials-and-appeals-in-aca-marketplace-plans-in-2023/

Loeb, N., & Loeb, N. (2020, December 8). *Four Little-Known Facts About Lewy Body Dementia - Lewy Body Dementia Resource Center.* Lewy Body Dementia Resource Center - Bringing awareness and supporting with love. https://lewybodyresourcecenter.org/four-little-known-facts-about-lewy-body-dementia

Luscombe, B. (2024, July 18). *People Still Misunderstand Trauma, Says 'Body Keeps the Score' Author Bessel van der Kolk.* TIME. https://time.com/6998595/bessel-van-der-kolk-trauma-profile

Medical examiner reveals how Gene Hackman and his wife died. (2025, March 8). [Video]. NBC News. https://www.nbcnews.com/news/us-news/officials-share-update-mystery-deaths-gene-hackman-wife-rcna195281

National Institute on Aging. (2021, August 24). *The dangers of polypharmacy and the case for deprescribing in older adults.* www.nia.nih.gov. Retrieved February 2, 2025, from https://www.nia.nih.gov/news/dangers-polypharmacy-and-case-deprescribing-older-adults

Near-Death experiences. (2021, January 18). Psychology Today. https://www.psychologytoday.com/intl/basics/near-death-experiences

Rejection Sensitive Dysphoria (RSD). (2024, May 1). Cleveland Clinic. https://my.clevelandclinic.org/health/diseases/24099-rejection-sensitive-dysphoria-rsd

Shaw, I. (2024, October 17). *'Revolutionary' new laser test could detect dementia in just 5 minutes – years before symptoms set in. . .* The Irish Sun. https://www.thesun.ie/health/14021224/new-dementia-five-munite-test-laser-before-symptoms

Somatic self care. (n.d.). Office of Well-Being. https://www.hopkinsmedicine.org/office-of-well-being/connection-support/somatic-self-care

The body keeps the score. (n.d.). Bessel Van Der Kolk, MD. https://www.besselvanderkolk.com/resources/the-body-keeps-the-score

Valtonen, J., & Karrasch, M. (2020). *Polypharmacy-induced cognitive dysfunction and discontinuation of psychotropic medication: a neuropsychological case report.* Therapeutic advances in psychopharmacology, 10, 2045125320905734. https://doi.org/10.1177/2045125320905734

Vinkers, C. H., Kupka, R. W., Penninx, B. W., Ruhé, H. G., van Gaalen, J. M., van Haaren, P. C. F., Schellekens, A. F. A., Jauhar, S., Ramos-Quiroga, J. A., Vieta, E., Tiihonen, J., Veldman, S. E., Veling, W., Vis, R., de Wit, L. E., & Luykx, J. J. (2024). *Discontinuation of psychotropic medication: a synthesis of evidence across medication classes.* Molecular psychiatry, 29(8), 2575–2586. https://doi.org/10.1038/s41380-024-02445-4

What are frontotemporal disorders? Causes, symptoms, and treatment. (2021, July 30). https://www.nia.nih.gov/. Retrieved February 1, 2025, from https://www.nia.nih.gov/health/frontotemporal-disorders/what-are-frontotemporal-disorders-causes-symptoms-and-treatment

What is lewy body dementia? Causes, symptoms, and treatments. (2021, July 29). https://www.nia.nih.gov/. Retrieved February 1, 2025, from https://www.nia.nih.gov/health/lewy-body-dementia/what-lewy-body-dementia-causes-symptoms-and-treatments

What's driving the demand for SLP's? | AMN Healthcare. (2022, October 18). https://www.amnhealthcare.com/amn-insights/news/speech-language-pathologists/

Wikipedia contributors. (2025, January 10). *Terminal lucidity*. Wikipedia. https://en.wikipedia.org/wiki/Terminal_lucidity

Printed in Dunstable, United Kingdom